MW00657033

The Candida Chronicles

A Manual for Candida Yeast Infections

Updated 2019 Edition

by

Michael Biamonte CCN.

Disclaimer and Terms of Use: The Author has strived to be as accurate and complete as possible in the creation of this book, notwithstanding the fact that he does not warrant or represent at any time that the contents within are accurate due to the rapidly changing nature of the Internet. While all attempts have been made to verify information provided in this publication, the Author assumes no responsibility for errors, omissions, or contrary interpretation of the subject matter herein. Any perceived slights of specific persons, peoples, or organizations are unintentional. In practical advice books, like anything else in life, there are no guarantees of income made. Readers are cautioned to rely on their own judgment about their individual circumstances to act accordingly. This book is not intended for use as a source of legal, business, accounting or financial advice. All readers are advised to seek services of competent professionals in the legal, business, accounting, and finance fields.

Acknowledgements

To my wife, Marie Tesa Biamonte, who always stood by me, believed in my abilities and who always contributed with her own wisdom, forethought and conviction that the truth be known.

To L. Ron Hubbard, who taught me how to think and how to interpret data.

To Robert Santoro, ND, who's own wisdom and insight inspired and guided me.

For my Father Michael Biamonte Sr. and my Uncle Charles Cumo, who set forth a dream for me.

And for my teacher, Dom Minasi, who helped contact and cultivate my abilities and creativeness.

Finally, for Mariska Hargitay: actress, activist and founder of the 'Joyful Heart Foundation.' She has inspired me; and, by her own actions, has shown me that helping our fellows is the goal expression of the artist's work.

Forward

By
Adam Banning

It was 1992 in New York City: I was 32 years old and was recently hired as a sales representative for a respected dietary supplement manufacturer. Our target market was healthcare practitioners who recommended vitamins, minerals, herbs, probiotics, and homeopathies to their patients. For six months I presented research on our formulas to some of the most interesting medical doctors, nutritionists, chiropractors, and naturopaths I had ever met. Then, on a very hot day at the end of July, I visited an office I'll never forget.

I took an overcrowded Number 6 train down to the City Hall station in Manhattan and walked two blocks south to Liberty Street for my first appointment of the day. I entered the office building and scanned the directory for the name of the doctor. A short middle eastern doorman walked up to me and said, "You looking for the Biamonte Center?" "How'd you know?", I responded. To which he only replied, "Sixth Floor," and then turned and walked back to his desk.

I took the elevator up to the sixth floor in search of the office of Dr. Michael Biamonte. I walked into his office, told the receptionist, Danielle, that I was the doctor's 9 am appointment and sat down in the waiting room. I was 15 minutes early, so I started reading one of the doctor's brochures on Candida and checked out the many pictures of celebrities on the walls. Could these all be patients? Many of the pictures were signed with rave reviews about, "Doctor B."

At 9 am, and I mean EXACTLY 9 am, Dr. Michael Biamonte opened the door of his office, looked at me with a warm and knowing smile, and said, "You must be Adam from Metagenics. Come on in."

He lead me into his exam room where there were tall stacks of studies on his big wooden desk and complex medical charts all over the walls. He sat behind his desk, and I took a seat in front. Then the first thing that came out of his mouth was, "So,,,, What do you know about Candida?"

"Like Vaginal Infections?" I asked. To which he responded, "Just the tip of the iceberg."

Dr. Biamonte graciously spent nearly an hour of his time educating me on the public health threat related to Candida infections and on his unique and well documented methods of treatment. After showing me dozens of peer reviewed journal studies on the subject and teaching me how to read a number of medical and biochemical charts in his office, he sent me on my way with a recommended reading list and a great deal of insight into health and the wonders of the human body.

Over the past 23 years, I've consulted with "Doctor B" for his insights that have helped me and thousands of his patients overcome major health challenges. Now he has written the "Candida Chronicles" to help millions more.

Table of Contents

Preface

HOW YOUR INSURANCE COVERAGE CAN MAKE YOU SICKER

Unfortunately, many of the cutting-edge treatments and cutting-edge doctors are not covered by insurance. When you read about illnesses like Candida, Epstein Barr, Lyme disease, Autism, Neurotransmitter imbalances, Elevated Cortisol syndromes, and Mercury toxicity you will be quick to find out that the doctors who are most qualified to treat these problems are not covered by your insurance plan or company. Often, these doctors do not take insurance as full payment because the insurance companies don't cover them in the first place.

There are some exceptions like Travelers Insurance, Aetna, and United Health Care which -- in the past -- have offered policies that cover holistic healing. About a third of American adults use some form of complementary or alternative medicine, according to reports by the National Center for Health Statistics. We spend more than $30 billion a year out of pocket on everything from fish oil supplements to acupuncture. However, despite those billions of dollars spent annually on alternative medicine and complementary treatments, most of these services are not currently covered by the majority of health insurers. The majority of those out-of-pocket expenses -- $14.7 billion in the most recent year studied --went to complementary and integrative health practitioners such as chiropractors, acupuncturists, and massage therapists. We spent another $12.8 billion on natural products and $2.7 billion on - care approaches, such as wellness books and homeopathic medicines.

Despite billions of dollars spent annually on alternative medicine, most of these services are not currently covered by the majority of health insurers: health insurance companies still regard most alternative techniques with uncertainty.

This lack of coverage often drives people to seek medical help from practitioners who will take their insurance but who are not actually qualified to address the patient's condition. For example, if you had a problem that was improved by the correct diet and nutritional supplements, would you rather see a clinical nutritionist who has over 2000 hours of study and certification in that field or a medical doctor who, on average, studies a total of 15 hours of nutrition as it relates to newborns and the elderly?

An analogy would be if someone gave you a food card that covered the majority of your food expenses, but the only place you were able to eat at was McDonalds. You might use that food card occasionally, but if that was the only place you ate (simply because it was cheap and covered by that food card), you would get sick and overweight. It would be bad for you, and you would use your own money to pay for more nutritious options.

When it comes to your health, you should be asking the question, "Is this doctor qualified and competent with a track record of success?" Not, "Does my insurance cover this?"

The neglect of insurance system to cover practitioners trained in alternative medicine will force you to seek the WRONG care and not get well!

Chapter 1

My Story

Years ago when I first started to practice as a nutritionist, I met a group of men who were developing a computer software program that could simulate all the functions and pathways of the human body. These fellows had backgrounds in systems analysis, engineering, nutrition, physiology, and aerospace physiology. Most of the group were employed by Grumman Aerospace and had participated in the development of life supports systems in the LEM (the craft that actually landed on the moon) or other such endeavors. The goal of their current project was to create software that could analyze basic blood, urine, and mineral tests and then use that data to identify nutritional errors and deficiencies and to indicate to professionals which vitamins, minerals, diets, and other factors would optimize or correct the ide problems.

I worked with the team for many years helping them to develop this software. I still remember all of those Sundays that I would climb aboard the Long Island Railroad to go way out east on Long Island to meet with them and help build the system. This system was and still is called "Biocybernetics Inc.", a name that refers to the study of how the body regulates itself. While I was using the system myself on the various clients who came to me for nutritional advice, I noticed that about 25 – 30 percent of the people who followed the vitamin and diet recommendation provided by the software program had "weird" responses. While most people who followed the software recommendations improved as expected, some couldn't tolerate the vitamins, and their condition worsened. I took it upon myself to discover what was different about these people, and it turned out that many had long histories of allergies and food and chemical sensitivities.

At the time I thought "Candida problems" were another fad invented by “flaky avocado eating health fanatics.” After several months of studying what was unique to about the people for whom the software recommendations did not work, I concluded that it was some type of microorganism. The computer analysis indicated that all of these people had lots of microorganism wastes being handled by their organs of elimination. I had some of these people tested by their own doctors for viruses, bacterial infections, Lyme, HIV, herpes and other such chronic conditions. While most of the patients came up negative for these conditions, what they did come up positive for was Candida and parasites!

“Oh no!” I thought “Was I wrong?” Could the flaky health fanatics be right? Was there something to avocado and sprout sandwiches that I was missing?”

I began to study the effects of Candida and determined that the patients who were having negative reactions to the software-created programs did, indeed, have Candida. It seemed logical that before they could go back on the computer-generated program we have to eliminate Candida from their systems. I sent these patients to their medical doctors. Some of the doctors said that they didn’t know how to treat it; while others said I was wrong because only AIDS patients have Candida; and still others tried to treat it, but the patients relapsed quickly.

I also amazed at how many doctors were not only in the dark about Candida but were also violently against the idea that it could be true that their patients could be harboring the organism. Some doctors would become hysterical and angry at the very mention of Candida. This reaction really got my attention, because for any group highly trained professionals to become so adamant that the results were wrong and so sure that their patients could not have Candida, I just had to think there was some fire behind all their smoke!” Then one day it occurred to me: If I was a medical doctor, and I gave people antibiotics to take every day, and if antibiotics can cause this yeast to grow out of control, and then it makes these people chronically sick for years and years and they never know quite what's wrong, would I run around saying, "Oh yeah you're right! It's all true! Candida is just what all those popular books say it is, and I cause it in people every time I write a script for an antibiotic. Yeah, sure, sue me!"

That's when I realized that medical doctors had a vested interest in maintaining the belief that Candida is a myth. So I sent my clients to alternative medical doctors who practice nutritional medicine. These doctors were eager to help. However their programs didn't always work. They did much better than the mainstream group of doctors but sooner or later too many of the patients relapsed.

That got me mad because it was wrecking my research! So I started to study this yeast. The more I studied about Candida, the more I saw that no one had a real comprehensive program to handle it. There were no standard protocols. Methods to treat it were as different and as many as there are stars in the sky.

I approached Candida from the roots up. I studied how it grew, what it ate, how it reproduced: every facet of its life cycle. I looked at anything that could help reduce Candida. And most of all, I really listened to my own patients. To how it affected them and to what seemed to help them feel better or make it worse. Then, after three years, I came across the work of Scott J. Gregory who had written a book called "The Holistic Protocol for the Immune System." I found that his work was very similar to my own conclusions. I called him often by telephone and ran by him many of my conclusions and proposed programs and the Candida testing I was researching.

By this point most of the Candida patients were getting well and staying that way. Had I slain the beast of yeast? No, not yet because quite a few would still relapse. So I studied what was different about those people. I found the causes of relapse over the years until 80 – 90 percent of those on my program stayed free of Candida. Those who continued to relapse usually didn't follow the program or had some much stress in their life that nothing could work.

In the late 1980's, The C.W. POST College radio station invited me to come on and debate with a very high-powered MD about Candida. I accepted. I had a good idea of what I was in for and rather than going on the show and having a shouting match, I came up with a better strategy. I came on the show with six medical books from which I had obtained a lot of my own data on Candida. I put paper clips in all the pages that had the data. The radio host introduced the medical doctor first. He went through his very impressive credentials. Then he bellowed out that "THERE'S NO SUCH THING AS CANDIDA." THIS IS ALL QUACKERY TO DECEIVE AND TRICK THE PUBLIC BY CHIROPRACTORS."

He went on and on: "It's not true! People being treated for Candida are not addressing their real underlying conditions, which could be cancer, and they could die! And that is why all the nutritionists and chiropractors are quacks!" This went on for 10 minutes or so non-sto. He never came up for air!

Then it was my turn, and, like a lawyer, I asked him if he could identify the books I had on the table. He said yes. I asked if he knew of these books personally. He said they were standard medical texts used in any good medical school. I asked if someone could consider this information reliable and trustworthy. he said of course and was now getting uncomfortable., he wanted me to get to the point, but didn't know that "the point" was aimed right at his heart. "So," I asked "if someone reads something in these books you would say that it would be sound, authoritative scientific data and true! Is that right?" "Yes, yes" he said. "I don't see the point to this. What are you trying to prove?"

I then picked up the first book and began simply reading what it had to say about Candida that completely contradicted his entire "opening argument." I continued with the next book and then the next book. Everything I was reading from the very books he had sanctioned was flying in the teeth of his all argument. I read page after page of what symptoms it could cause, how antibiotics, birth control pills, estrogen medications, and steroids could cause the condition. The host of the show almost lost control of his bladder he started laughing so hard! I continued for six minutes just reading and quoting.

Then suddenly he stood up as if he was going to pound on the top of my head with the bottom of his fist and grabbed the book out of my hand. "See here and give me that!" He then started flipping pages like a mad man. "You're twisting this! I don't mean Candida doesn't exist, I mean that is doesn't make people as ill as you people say it does!" With that I picked up the last book. "Well it says here that "if not treated it can lead to allergies, dermatitis, it's linked to Autism and a host of digestive disorders, it's right here in the book that you said was trustworthy!" He then stared into the book with a glazed look on his face, "But they don't really mean that in everyone!" "They don't mean that.. I tell you! It's not true! You don't know what you're talking about!"

At this point he stormed out of the studio never to return, probably to buy gun and shoot the authors of the medical books I had brought in! Was this David and Goliath on college radio?

And that is why your doctor may not like this book. A lot has happened since the late 1980's. There have been many books written on Candida, and it's much more widely accepted that it is the culprit that it is. There have been thousands of studies and papers from many sources. So beware of any doctor who says, "THERE'S NO SUCH THING AS CANDIDA!"

Chapter 2

Candida: History, Causes, Effects on Human Health. Where Does It Live? What Does It Eat?

In September 1972, two founders of the Federation of Feminist Women's Health Centers, Carol Downer and Colleen Wilson, were arrested for allegedly practicing medicine without a license. Their Los Angeles Self-Help Clinic was raided by the California Department of Consumer Affairs and the Board of Medical Examiners who apparently had nothing better to do. The Self-Help Clinic presented the local medical establishment with competition. Concerned with the potential loss of revenue for the local physicians, one doctor, three uniformed police, and several plainclothes investigators confiscated four truckloads of supplies and equipment in order to shut down operations of the women-controlled clinic. The reason for the arrest? Downer had inserted yogurt into the vagina of a women's center staff member. The trial became known as the "Great Yogurt Conspiracy" and was a crucial turning point in the women's health movement. Downer was found not guilty by arguing that applying yogurt as a home remedy for an ordinary yeast infection is not practicing medicine. The verdict reinforced women's control over their own bodies and established that at-home methods of self-care are, indeed, lawful.

The Right of Self-Help and Self-Care

The feminist movement fostered Consciousness Raising (CR) groups -- small friendship networks of women who gathered to share their life stories and to create change in their lives. Carol Downer brought a plastic speculum into her CR group, and the group began to focus on self-help vaginal and cervical self-exams. Later, she and the others founded the LA Self-Help clinic to share what they had learned with other women.

These self-help groups flourished around the country as women investigated what was, for them, new territory in women's health. They researched natural, home remedies and discovered useful tools to self-care, such as yogurt to combat yeast infections. These groups spread the knowledge to other women and together they demanded simpler, easier alternative treatments to common conditions such as yeast.

The Battle with the FDA

"Self-helpers" used their knowledge to critically examine the medical establishment. Why were women relying on healthcare providers for things they could do themselves? Many of these women began political work, using their new knowledge to advocate for women's healthcare more generally. These activists had a decades-long battle with the Food and Drug Administration, pharmaceutical companies, and medical care providers preceding the FDA's approval of yeast medications for over-the-counter (OTC) sale. For decades after the Great Yogurt Conspiracy, women were still required to make and pay for an appointment at the gynecologist, have a pelvic exam, and fill a prescription to cure this easily recognized and easily treated condition. Women had been spending millions of dollars a year for care of problems they could easily manage themselves.

Yet, when women's activism finally paid off with FDA approval for OTC sale of yeast creams, the cost of a one-time dose ranged from $13 to $20. Further, there are even easier to use prescription methods available now, created after the standard treatment became available OTC. In order to obtain these simpler and easier methods, effective in just a fraction of the time the older medications take to work, women must still see a doctor. Drug companies, male-dominated healthcare institutions, and federal health policy-makers control women's healthcare: what medications are available, what the standard of care is for women's health problems, what health conditions are investigated and who can treat women. Yeast treatment is just one item on a long list of issues in women's healthcare, such as HIV/AIDS, breast cancer, and heart disease, that has been overlooked and mishandled by those in control. The journey yeast medications have taken shows that, evidently, this control will not be easily surrendered.

Over-The-Counter Remedies

The OTC medication manufacturers have been advertising aggressively since the FDA approval. Today, it is as common to see TV ads for Monistat or Gyne-Lotrimin as it is for breakfast cereal. These brands, as well as the three or four others in the running, provide a chemical neutralization for the build-up of vaginal yeast. They are creams inserted with an applicator, usually at bedtime, over the course of 7 days. During the treatment, a woman is supposed to avoid baths and sexual intercourse.

What You Can Try at Home for Starters

Many women use non-medical methods for treating yeast, because the cost of over-the-counter methods is high, because they are unimpressed with OTC methods, or simply because they prefer more natural methods. The following is a partial list of at-home methods that may be helpful. If your condition has been chronic, these may not work, and you should seek a doctor who can guide you through the programs in this book.

- Insert unpasteurized, plain yogurt overnight. Be sure the yogurt you use contains live cultures of acidophilus or lactobacillus (it will say so on the label). Insert at least two tablespoons daily. Insert at night and wear a pad. Repeat for three to seven nights until symptoms disappear. Here are some tips for getting it in there. Yogurt can be inserted with an empty tampon inserter, vaginal cream inserter, or a turkey baster (the baster works best).

Symptoms could be relieved within 24 hours. Douching with yogurt and water can help, too. It also helps to eat a lot of yogurt. Make sure the yogurt contains acidophilus and bifidus cultures. Health food stores are the best choice.

- "Paint" the vagina, cervix (you'll need a speculum) and vulva (outside area including the labia or "lips" of vagina) with gentian violet. It stains, so you'll want to wear a pad. This usually works after one treatment. Biocidin is an example of a gentian product.
- Insert a garlic suppository. Carefully peel one clove of garlic. Wrap in gauze and insert into the vagina. Leave in for up to twelve hours. Repeat as necessary. It also helps to eat a lot of garlic.
- Drink cranberry juice. Unsweetened is best. Sweetened juice may feed the yeast and make it spread. Try a cranberry concentrate from the health food store.
- Insert potassium sorbate. This is used in home beer-making and can be found at wine-making stores. Dip a cotton tampon into a 3 percent solution (15 grams of potassium sorbate in one pint of water) and insert into the vagina at night. Remove in the morning.
- Drink or eat acidophilus. It is available in powder or capsules in health food stores or found in some milk and yogurt products. (Read the label; some dairy products have added acidophilus.)
- Douche with a vinegar/water solution: one tablespoon of vinegar to one quart of water, once a day. This is especially effective when used with yogurt suppositories.
- Nix the feminine deodorant sprays. No soap, nylon bathing suits, or pantyhose without a cotton crotch. Wear only cotton or nothing at all. Hot, moist environments incubate yeast.

- Insert two acidophilus capsules into your vagina daily. Lactobacilli such as acidophilus are natural residents of a healthy vagina. They prevent overgrowths of yeast. (They also turn milk into yogurt.) Adding lactobacilli vaginally stops yeast from growing and creates copious amounts of lubrication.
- If the yeast is persistent, and you experience chronic or repeated overgrowths, then your sexual partner may need to be treated as well. Have him soak his penis in yogurt or diluted apple cider for five minutes daily to kill the yeast living in or on the glans; this way he won't keep reinfecting you.
- If neither acidophilus nor yogurt cure the yeast, you need to re-acidify your vagina. Boric acid is the most efficient, and you can purchase it in the drug store. Dilute it one teaspoon to one cup of warm water and mini-douche daily with the barrel of a syringe or use a diaphragm jelly inserter which can be bought at the pharmacy without having to buy the jelly. Do not use this method if your skin is raw or broken and discontinue if an irritation develops. This is wet and messy, but boric acid is anti-bacterial and will cleanse some non-specific vaginitis as well.
- Apple cider vinegar douches (two tablespoons vinegar to a pint of warm water) are very effective. Even though yeast flourishes in an acidic environment, there is something in vinegar that inhibits its growth. Vinegar can also inhibit the growth of bacteria and trichomonas by establishing the proper acidity (pH) for the proliferation of "good" bacteria. Do not douche for longer than 10 days.

Regular douching should be discouraged. The vagina is a self-cleaning environment, so routine douching should not be necessary and could make your vagina too alkaline. Women who douche more than three times a month are four to five times more likely to have rampant yeast.

Non-Specific Bacterial Vaginitis

Non-specific vaginitis is bacterial and is characterized by burning and itching, usually with a discharge, odor, sometimes a rash and painful intercourse. It is probably a good idea to visit your local midwife or nurse practitioner and have her check it out under a microscope to see what kind of bacteria you are dealing with. To eliminate a mild bacterial infection, do the following:

- Garlic -- Insert a peeled clove of garlic high up into your vagina, being sure to push it all the way up to the cervix (which feels like the tip of your nose) every night for a week. Garlic is well known for its antibiotic properties, but you may walk around smelling vaguely like a pizza.
- Betadine (povidone-iodine) suppositories and douches are available in drug stores and help cure nonspecific vaginitis. Wear a pad to control staining.
- Tee tree oil or grapefruit seed extracts are now sold as douches. They can be very effective in killing yeast and bacteria. Look for them in your health food stores.
- Lastly, as with all of menopause, you are more likely to be troubled with vaginal complaints if your adrenals have been exhausted by overuse of coffee, cigarettes, alcohol and white sugar. See a nutritionist or doctor who can help you repair your adrenal glands.

Women experiencing persistent vaginal yeast overgrowth who are using a cervical cap or diaphragm need to wash and dry it well after use. Some women have found relief from tenacious conditions with the "sucking air" method of douching. In a bathtub, a woman can insert yogurt, vinegar, or another remedy. Lying on her back, hands at her side and palms down, she can bring her feet back over her head. This action causes the vagina to balloon out and pulls the vinegar or yogurt all the way in to fill the vagina and get every fold of skin.

Systemic yeast is a system-wide infection/overgrowth throughout the body. It requires dramatic changes in diet and long-term attention to avoiding things that encourage yeast to grow.

Yeast and HIV

Having a yeast condition might increase your susceptibility to contracting HIV since vaginal irritation may allow easier passage of the virus into the bloodstream. For years, women's health advocates worked to demonstrate that the common perception of HIV and AIDS was based on men's experiences, and it is now recognized that nearly-constant yeast overgrowth can be a marker of HIV infection in women. The immune system suppression from HIV can cause an imbalance in the vagina's chemistry, resulting in persistent yeast overgrowth.

Douching

The vagina is a self-cleaning organ and, as such, does not need "washing." In fact, regular douching can be harmful because it creates an upset in the normal vaginal pH. In a healthy vagina, douching can actually cause a yeast infection if it kills that friendly bacteria!

- Manufacturers of douches, deodorants, scented tampons, soaps, and perfumes would have us believe the vagina is dirty. In order to sell their products they must make us believe women's bodies are naturally unclean and have unpleasant odors. However, a healthy vagina has a pleasant, lightly musky odor, and chemicals like those found in many products can mask changes in that odor which may signal an infection. The chemicals in these products can also be harmful, by irritating the skin, mucous membrane, and the pH balance of the vagina. Unless it is used as a method for treating problems such as yeast overgrowth, douching is unnecessary.

The Answer to Your Vaginal Infection is Not Political: My Approach And Perspectives

Many women with whom I consult have been in and out of their doctor's office with chronic yeast infections without finding out why or what to do to get rid of it once and for all. And there is an answer. If you have been told that the itching and burning you felt were not really there, that was false. If a doctor accused you of doing unsanitary things to cause your infections, it is due his lack of understanding and his inability to confront the problem. You may have noticed other strange symptoms, like reactions to foods and drinks, mood changes, extreme fatigue, a foggy lack of concentration, depression, and many other symptoms during a vaginal flare up. If a doctor told you they have nothing to do with each other, he was wrong. The odds are, most of what you suspected on your own about the whole subject of your vaginal infections is true. Let us first understand what is normal and what is not.

What is Normal?

It is considered normal for a small amount of white or grayish semi-solid material to be passed from the vaginal opening. This is the result of the normal breakdown and repair of cells in the cervix and the vagina. A watery or mucous-like secretion from the cervix should occur in response to sexual stimulation. During ovulation, the discharge may be bloodied. This is normal.

What is Not Normal

A white, creamy-white, or yellow mucous-like discharge indicates an infection in either the vagina, cervix, endo-cervix, or endometrium. The discharge may be frothy and cottage cheese-like in the case of many yeast-type infections. A very foul smelling discharge is common in bacterial infections or when tampons or contraceptive devices are left neglected. A watery mucous-less discharge sometimes occurs in malignancy of the upper genital tract or from radiation therapy. Sometimes it can be caused by abnormal narrowing of the cervix or endo-cervix.

During childhood or after menopause the vaginal mucus is thin and lacks proper amounts of friendly bacteria which inhibit the growth of the infection-causing bacteria. Also the mucous lining carries an immune-boosting substance which protects against infections. If this was all there was to the story, women in their active reproduction years would not be plagued with the vaginal infections.

In adults, the vaginal discharge is mostly caused by an infection in the lower reproductive tract. Trichomonas, Candida, gardnenella, E. coli, staphylococci, streptococci, and intestinal parasites are common causes. Other venereal infections may also cause the problem. Lower estrogen levels have been known to promote the growth of streptococci, staphylococci, coil-form bacilli, and diphtheriods and may cause chronic vaginal infections.

Candida infection is of course more common today due to the use of antibiotics, birth control pills, and chemical preparations. Years ago it was thought to occur only in diabetic and pregnant women. However, due to the incorrect treatment of vaginal yeast infections with antibiotics and cortisone, and due to the widespread use of oral contraceptives which stimulate the overgrowth of yeasts, Candida has risen to be a household word and the subject of many books besides this one! Candida is also called monilia, although the term is rarely used.

Vaginal Yeast Infection

A vaginal yeast infection may begin with an external itching and/or redness or swelling of the vulva. At times the burning and pain can be so bed that it interferes with walking. A whitish, non-bloody discharge either light or heavy, watery to cottage cheese-like is common. It will smell like vinegar or yeast. Pain during intercourse is a very common sign. If you have chronic yeast infections, the symptoms will worsen one week to 10 days prior to menses.

Candida is a sneaky organism. As described in other sections of this book, it can change form from a yeast to a fungus. As a fungus, it grows into a plant-like structure, digging into your cells to find food. Women have described it as "having plants growing in there." In its fungal form, Candida is sometimes less noticeable but will cause hundreds of symptoms not generally thought of as being connected to a yeast infection. In the yeast form it is easier to control. Antibiotics may reduce the infections for a short time, only to have it come back with a vengeance.

Many doctors have failed to diagnose Candida due to the fact that it often is found with other bacteria. When Candida is present, other infection-causing bacteria have been known to grow and cause infections. Studies show that injecting animals with small amounts of Candida along with small amounts of staph or strep will cause a huge infection. When animals are given much larger doses of staph or strep with no Candida, infections or symptoms were much less severe. This may have happened to you. If so, proper diagnosis was missed. The medical profession is so lost on how to handle this problem that on television we now see ads for creams and other anti-yeast medication. This is their way of trying to cope with the floods of women who are not permanently helped and, of course, the "yogurt conspiracy."

Proper treatment and diagnosis of Candida Albicans is essential in helping you. You can get better and get rid of the condition. But it can take many months or years. Why? Because Candida can travel through your body. Candida can 'nest' in the bowel but go on vacation in other parts of your body and may take up residence there. When it returns home it will set up its nest again. Also Candida cells can bury themselves deep into the cells of the bowel, and enough of them will remain to resume their lives and your discomfort once the cleansing is over.

I have found after five years of getting moderate success with other approaches, that the approaches described in this book make the most sense. Since I have obtained excellent results with chronic yeast infections (and other problems of this type) in patients who have been to every practitioner I have ever heard of and are still relapsing, no one will dare argue that this is not the fastest and best route to take. Mainstream medicine has only creams and toxic, potentially damaging drugs to offer. Most will harm you before they totally kill your infection. However, since mainstream medicine knows nothing about intestinal cleansing, vitamins, or immune-stimulating herbs, their patients will never get well. If they do, I would consider it a fluke.

The key to eliminating vaginal yeast infections is to stop treating just the vaginal yeast infection. A paper printed in "The Journal of the American Medical Association" in 1977 stated: "Vaginal candidiasis does not occur naturally without infection of C. Albicans within the large bowel and that a cure is not likely as long as the vagina remains the only treatment target."

To really handle the vaginal yeast infection, you must destroy not only the yeast in the vaginal area, but also the intestinal overgrowth of yeast. It is the intestinal overgrowth of yeast that makes you more susceptible to the vaginal problem.

It is an easy jaunt from the rectal area into the vaginal region for yeast. While yeasts do not have legs, feet, wheels, or other modes of transportation, they can get to the vaginal area easily by transfer from toilet paper that gets tiny yeast cells on it as you wipe after a bowel movement. Or, as gas is expelled in flatulence (or "farting"), yeast cells can "ride the wind" into or about the vaginal area. Once in the vaginal area, it is possible for the cells to grow into an infection if the immune system is weak, if there is a lack of friendly bacteria, or the pH is too alkaline.

Overgrowth of intestinal yeast will weaken and stress the immune response. This makes body more susceptible to having the smaller vaginal area become overrun by yeasts. If the intestinal area is overgrown with yeast, this means that much of the 40-foot-long small intestine and the 6- to 8-foot-long colon has yeast overgrowth. This places a significant strain on the immune system and can allow vaginal overgrowth simply because the immune system is being suppressed by the intestinal yeast.

The intestinal tract is literally the nest when it comes to yeasts and Candida in the body. Handling the intestinal yeast, or nest, relieves the immune system of quite a burden. Having this burden released frees up the "troops" to allow them to fight in the much smaller battleground of the vaginal area!

Candida and What Causes It

Candida is a normal member of the total population of micro(small) organisms in your intestines. The better question is what causes Candida overgrowth since it is the overgrowth of Candida that causes symptoms. I have seen people with high levels of "overgrowth" have a few symptoms and others with lower levels have really bad symptoms. The person with the high level can sometimes fight it off and detoxify the waste products of Candida faster than person who is feeling horrible from a lower level of overgrowth. As you will read later many factors affect Candida and your body's response to it.

The true causes of Candida overgrowth are not a mystery. They are also not the same for each individual. Some people have Candida due to a combination of causes. To begin with, let's look at the true causes and discuss each.

1. ANTIBIOTICS: Antibiotics are a common cause of Candida. Antibiotics destroy both harmful bacteria and good bacteria. When antibiotics destroy friendly bacteria, it gives the Candida a chance to begin to multiply. Anyone who has been treated with antibiotics for acne, major dental work, or any condition where antibiotic use has been more frequent than one course of 7-10 days is a prime Candidate for Candida overgrowth.

2. BIRTH CONTROL PILLS OR DEVICES: Oral birth control pills are mostly the hormone estrogen. Supplemental estrogen in the synthetic form has been found to promote the growth of yeast. Several years ago the Great Smokies Medical lab published studies showing that the hormones can affect intestinal bacteria. A common compliant of women on birth control pills is yeast infection. The copper IUD is another possible yeast promoter. It has been observed by David Watts Ph.D. that copper promotes the growth of yeast. Often copper IUD users develop excessive levels of copper in their tissues. Excess copper can depress the adrenal, thyroid, and immune systems of the body. This can make it more difficult for the body to resist yeast.

3. EXCESSIVE STRESS AND ELEVATED CORTISOL: Stress can cause yeast growth for several reasons. Stress causes the release of hormone called CORTISOL . Cortisol can depress the immune system and also raise blood sugar. The elevation in blood sugar can give feed the yeast cells, allowing them to grow quickly. The depression in immune function will leave the body defenseless against the sudden elevation in yeast. These two reactions tend to happen together as cortisol goes up. This is the exact reason why stress causes Candida. Cortisol can be addicting to the body. It raises sugar and relieves inflammation. There have been a few studies that show the body can become addicted to it and will try to keep it

elevated. There are several simple nutrients that help lower cortisol levels back to normal by telling the nervous system to relax.

4. TAP WATER CONSUMPTION: Common tap water is high in chlorine which has been found to destroy friendly intestinal bacteria. This will allow Candida to grow as covered earlier.

5. PARASITES AND INTESTINAL WORMS; Parasites and intestinal worms are more common than anyone would think. Some researchers have estimated that over 85 percent of all people living in North America and Canada have parasites. Parasites can be large worm-like creatures or small microscopic organisms. Either type destroys friendly bacteria in the intestines making yeast over growth possible.

6. CONSTIPATION; Constipation can be caused by Candida. However constipation can also lead to Candida. If a person does not have Candida and then becomes constipated for any reason, Candida may begin to grow. A digestive tract which is constipated is slow moving and becomes very alkaline. Candida thrives in an alkaline environment. The more alkaline the digestive tract, the happier the Candida becomes. It does not matter what causes the constipation. Constipation for any reason can easily cause Candida.

7. DRUGS AND ALCOHOL; Excess alcohol can directly destroy friendly bacteria and allow yeast to grow. Beer can be a particular problem and not because of the yeast, but because of its maltose content. Maltose is a sugar that is derived from malt. Malt sugar is very potent and can feed yeast cells very quickly. People with Candida also tend to develop allergies to all yeast products whether the yeast is healthy or not. This does not mean that hard spirits or wine in excess are any safer. Alcohol should always be used in moderation. Drugs can also cause yeast overgrowth particularly if they disturb the digestive system. Any medication or drug that can cause a gastrointestinal side effect may cause yeast growth by disturbing friendly bacteria.

8. HYPOTHYROID: Low thyroid is very common in cases of Candida. The thyroid gland has an important effect on the immune system. Adequate thyroid function also helps the digestive system operate correctly. As pointed out earlier, lack of proper digestive secretions can cause reduction of friendly bacteria. Constipation is also common with low thyroid. Body temperature will drop if thyroid function is low. A drop in body temperature stops many different chemical reactions from taking place. Some of these chemical reactions stop Candida overgrowth.

9. IMMUNE DEFICIENCY: Any condition that results in a weakened immune system can bring about Candida. Most notable are AIDS and cancer. Candida can be considered a side effect of these more threatening illnesses.

10. HORMONAL IMBALANCE: It has been long recognized that an imbalance between estrogen and progesterone can be a causative factor in yeast overgrowth. In order to support friendly intestinal flora, adequate amounts of both hormones are needed. The Great Smokies Medical Lab published a paper several years ago that explained how these hormones are essential to the health of friendly bacteria. Any upset in this balance can cause yeast overgrowth. The hormonal imbalance must be corrected after the yeast has been reduced or relapse is sure to occur.

11. EXCESSIVE BOWEL CLEANSING; I am a firm believer in colonic irrigation and bowel cleansing. However, it does happen that one can overdo cleansing. If someone has an excessive amount of colonics without replacing friendly bifidus bacteria that lives in the colon, Candida may grow. This is a rare situation, but noteworthy.

12. DIABETES; This is the most difficult case to deal with. It is essential that the diabetes be addressed first and the blood sugar be brought under control. It is impossible to eliminate Candida while the blood sugar is high. There are specific herbs that are antifungal and have traditionally

been used to lower blood sugar. I developed this protocol two years ago and have used it with good results, but I feel that most people should go right on a diabetic protocol to lower their sugar before attempting any Candida elimination.

13. MERCURY, COPPER, and ARSENIC; These are the thee toxic metals that I have seen most frequently in the Candida patient. Many of the patients who come to me bring toxic metal tests of hair, stool, or urine from previous doctors. These are the three most common that I find elevated in the Candida patient. Each one deserves its own chapter on how it will cause Candida.

Health Concerns Related to Candida

Candida has been documented to release several types of toxins into the system. Among them are mycotoxins. As many as 1,000 compounds -- classifiable as mycotoxins -- were studied by the pharmacology industry as potential antibiotics in the 1930s and 1940s only to be discarded as being too toxic for higher life forms to be of value in treating bacterial diseases in humans. Little, if any of the discarded data was published. Yet, what these toxicity studies actually documented was the existence of a large number of fungal-derived toxins which cause serious target organ injury in various animal models. Obviously, in retrospect, what was being seen was the pathology produced by the mycotoxins. In order to understand this toxicity, one only has to look at what some of these mycotoxins, used as medications, cause in humans:

The mycotoxin cyclosporin used for transplantation causes cancer and arteriosclerosis, complete with hyperlipidemia, in ALL humans who have received it. Many others develop gout and other diseases. However, to place the matter in proper perspective, the study of such fungal metabolites gave us penicillin at the beginning and, quite later on, cyclosporine and the most potent immunosuppressant transplantation drug, lovastatin and the other statins which have revolutionized the treatment of hyperlipidemia and arteriosclerosis. The latter group is quite interesting in that they were initially developed as antifungal agents which just happened to have an effect in lowering blood levels of low density lipoproteins (commonly referred to as "bad cholesterol").

Mycotoxicoses are diseases caused by mycotoxins, secondary byproducts of molds. Although they occur more frequently in areas with a hot and humid climate favorable for the growth of molds, they can also be found in temperate zones. Exposure to mycotoxins is mostly by ingestion, but also occurs by skin and inhalation routes. Mycotoxicoses often remain unrecognized by medical professionals, except when large numbers of people are involved

Mycotoxins exert toxic effects on animals and humans. The toxic effect of mycotoxins on animal and human health is referred to as Mycotoxicoses, the severity of which depends on the toxicity of the mycotoxins, the extent of exposure, age and nutritional status of the individual affected, and possible effects of other chemicals or toxins to which the individual has been exposed.

The History of Mycotoxins

The effect of molds and fungi was known already in ancient times. In the 7th and 8th centuries BC, the festival "Robigalia" was established to honor the god Robigus, who had to be propitiated in order to protect grain and trees. It was celebrated on 25 April because that was the most likely time for crops to be attacked by rust or mildew. In the Middle Ages, outbreaks of ergotism caused by ergot alkaloids from Claviceps Purpurea reached epidemic proportions, mutilating and killing thousands of people in Europe. Ergotism was also known as ignis sacer (sacred fire) or St Anthony's fire, because at the time it was thought that a pilgrimage to the shrine of St. Anthony would bring relief from the intense burning sensation experienced. The victims of ergotism were exposed to the hallucinogen lysergic acid diethylamide (LSD) produced during the baking of bread made with ergot-contaminated wheat, as well as to other ergot toxins and hallucinogens. Suffers were also exposed to belladonna alkaloids from the mandragora apple that was used to treat ergotism.

While ergotism no longer has such important implications for public health, recent reports indicate that outbreaks of human Mycotoxicoses are still possible. Some Mycotoxicoses have disappeared owing to more rigorous hygiene measures. For example, citreoviridin-related malignant acute cardiac beriberi ("yellow rice disease" or shoshin-kakke disease in Japanese) has not been reported for several decades following the exclusion of moldy rice from the markets. Citreoviridin is a metabolic product of Penicillium citreonigrum, which grows readily on rice during storage after harvest, especially in the colder regions of Japan. Another Mycotoxicoses not seen for decades is alimentary toxic aleukia, common in the 1930s and 1940s in the USSR. This disease was caused by trichothecenes produced by Fusarium strains on unharvested grain.

General interest in mycotoxins rose in 1960 when a feed-related Mycotoxicoses called turkey X disease, which was later proved to be caused by aflatoxins, appeared in farm animals in England. Subsequently it was found that aflatoxins are hepatocarcinogens in animals and humans, and this stimulated research on mycotoxins. There is a long history of the use of certain molds in the production of cheese and salami and in the fermentation of beer and wine. Molds are also used in the production of drugs (antibiotics). The classification of mold metabolites as antibiotics or mycotoxins is based on their toxicity or beneficial effect in treating diseases. Some mold metabolites that were initially considered to be antibiotics (e.g. citrinin) were subsequently found to be highly toxic and are currently classified as toxins. Ergot alkaloids are still used, inter alia, in the treatment of Parkinson's Disease, as prolactin inhibitors and in cerebrovascular insufficiency, migraine treatment, venous insufficiency, thrombosis and embolisms, for the stimulation of cerebral and peripheral metabolism, in uterine stimulation, and as a dopaminergic agonist.

The toxic effects of mycotoxins (e.g. ochratoxins, fumonisins, zearalenone, etc.) are mostly known from veterinary practice. Mycotoxicoses, which can occur in both industrialized and developing countries, arise when environmental, social, and economic conditions combine with meteorological conditions (humidity, temperature) that favor the growth of molds.

The Nervous System

Candida produces other toxins that affect the nervous system. In 1978 C. Orian Truss M.D first began a series of publications that explained the mental and neurological effects of Candida. Truss also speculated on the relationship of Candida to repeated ear infections and learning problems in children. His reports chronicle the lives and treatment of several patients suffering with neurological illness that responded to Candida treatments.

Dr. William Shaw has been conducting important research on yeast and its effects on autistic individuals. He recently discovered unusual microbial metabolites in the urine of autistic children who responded remarkably well to anti-fungal treatments. Dr. Shaw and his colleagues observed a decrease in urinary organic acids as well as decreases in hyperactivity and self-stimulatory, stereotyped behavior and increases in eye contact, vocalization, and concentration.

Several years ago, I was fortunate enough to attend a seminar in which Bernard Rimland, Ph.D. of the Autism Research Institute spoke for several hours about the connection between Candida and autism. Dr.Rimland shared with us statistical data that he combined over many years. This data was compiled by having the parents of autistic children fill out a questionnaire that summarized the child's overall health and behavior. The questionnaire was repeated several months later. Of 208 cases in the study, 49 percent showed significant improvement and only 4 percent worsened on nystatin or ketoconzale(anti-fungals drugs). This was the best improvement: worsening ratio of any of the 31 drug treatments used, including Ritalin.

Chronic Fatigue Syndrome

William G Crook accurately describes the relationship between Candida and chronic fatigue syndrome (CFS) is his book, "Chronic Fatigue Syndrome and The Yeast Connection." Crook points out that women between the ages of 25 and 40 seem especially prone to "CFS." Why? It seems rather simple. This is the typical age span during which women menstruate. And a woman's hormones have a great impact on Candida!

Classic Chronic Fatigue Syndrome was originally thought to be caused by the Epstein Barr virus which is the virus that also causes Mononucleosis. However, CFS has branched out to include many disorders that result in "Chronic Fatigue." The original "model" of it being caused by a viral infection has been broadened coincidentally to the condition being reimbursable by insurance companies.

I have observed that 90 percent of Candida suffers describe or feel they have "chronic fatigue." Moreover, I feel that many times Candida is actually a "Mixed Infection Syndrome," where the Candida suffer or the viral suffer becomes host to several infections due to her weakened immunity. It is not unusual to find that the Candida suffer at one time has active viruses, parasites, and other infections along with Candida. In a sense, having any one of these makes you susceptible to the others.

Symptoms of Candida

Candida is capable of producing over 100 symptoms. This tends to make it extremely frustrating for anyone with this condition to be able to find out or to understand what is exactly wrong with them. Billions are spent each year on antibiotics, creams, nasal sprays, unnecessary hospital visits, operations, and antidepressants due to the ignorance and arrogance of the medical profession. It is written in their own journals that antibiotics can cause this condition, yet they continue to boldly prescribe them and are resentful when discussing their side effects

The symptoms of Candida are so confusing that even a practitioner who wants to know about it can be confused. Look over the list of all the possible symptoms Candida can cause, and you will see why I so firmly believe that by symptoms alone one can be misled into treating a "major symptom" and miss the true culprit.

SYMPTOMS OF CANDIDA

1 Intolerance of perfumes, odors, fumes, fabric shop odors and tobacco smoke.
2 Complaints that worsen in damp, muggy or moldy places.
3 Athletes' foot, jock itch, fungal infections on the skin or nails.
4 Craving for sugar, bread or alcohol.
5 Prostitis or vaginitis.
6 Diarrhea.
7 Constipation.
8 Abdominal distention, bloating or pain.
9 Gas or flatulence.
10 Rectal itching or rash.
11 Colic.
12 Diaper rash.
13 Vaginal itch, burning or persistent infections.
14 Kidney, bladder infections.
15 Cystitis (inflammation of the bladder with possible infection).
16 Sinus infections.
17 Joint pain or swelling.
18 Acne.
19 Hives.
20 Rashes.
21 Itching skin.
22 Eczema.
23 Psoriasis.
24 Loss of sex drive.
25 Impotence.
26 Fatigue.
27 Feeling drained.
28 Memory loss.
29 Feeling spaced out.

30 Numbness, burning or tingling.
31 Muscle aches.
32 Muscle pains.
33 Flu-like symptoms.
34 Endometriosis (irregular or painful menstruation).
35 Cramps or menstrual irregularities.
36 P.M.S.
37 Spots in front of eyes.
38 Erratic vision.
39 Drowsiness.
40 Irritability or jitteriness.
41 Mood swings.
42 Depression.
43 Suicidal feelings.
44 Headaches.
45 Hypoglycemia.
46 Feeling of swelling and tingling in the head.
47 Heartburn.
48 Indigestion.
49 Belching.
50 Intestinal gas.
51 Mucus in the stools.
52 Hemorrhoids.
53 Dry mouth.
54 Sores or blisters in the mouth
55 Bad breath.
56 Nasal congestion.
57 Nasal discharge.
58 Nasal itching.
59 Post nasal drip.
60 Sore or dry mouth.
61 Sore or dry throat.
62 Cough.
63 Pain or tightness in the chest.
64 Wheezing or shortness of breath.
65 Asthmatic symptoms.
66 Burning or itching eyes.
67 Burning on urination.
68 Ear pain.
69 Ear aches.
70 Ear discharges.
71 Painful intercourse.
72 Food allergies or food reactions.
73 Hay fever.
74 General allergies.
75 Thrush.
76 Hair loss.

As you can see, the symptoms are so varied that no one person has a set of symptoms identical to that of another person. The average Candida sufferer has 20 or more of these (while others have less and some have more). Many times they have given up on ever finding out what was wrong with them because all of these symptoms seem unrelated.

One patient spent seven days in the hospital, was wheeled from one examination room to another -- a grand tour of the hospital -- only to be told it was all in her head. She was charged over $6000.00 for that stay. Upon her release a stool analysis was done and Candida was found. In addition, all the Jell-O and the horrible hospital food worsened her symptoms.

Symptoms of Candida, regardless of what they are, can change due to different conditions. These conditions can change and then the symptoms will change. There are several factors that can change the symptoms. Some are under a person's control and some are not:

1. **Weather:** Hot, humid or muggy weather. Like any mold or fungus, heat and humidity help it grow and spread.
2. **Diet:** Symptoms can also vary according to one's diet. Sugar, alcohol, starches, fermented foods; sweets (even fruits) will increase symptoms by feeding the yeast organisms. This will cause them to grow and release more toxins which will produce symptoms.
3. **Stress:** Stress is key to triggering symptoms. It has long been recognized that stress plays a part in lowering the immune function of the body. The immune system is what tries to keep the yeast under control. Simply being over-worked, over-tired, or over-stressed will cause an increase in Candida and therefore its symptoms.
4. **Environment:** The environment in which one can play a big role if one is exposed to toxic metals, fumes, smoke, and pollution and is in direct contact with various chemicals. The immune system can become overloaded and therefore further dip, which will allow more yeast to grow.

If a person finds these conditions causing an increase in symptoms then there is a very good chance that Candida is present. The problem for Candida suffers is they may start to avoid foods that they have painstakingly found worsen their symptoms. The sufferers have unknowingly put themselves on the Candida diet, and they feel better. Then the weather changes. It becomes hot and humid, and some symptoms return along with the fatigue. Suffers conclude that the foods were not the answer, so they stop the diet. Now they feel worse again. Now summer ends and takes the heat and humidity with it. The sufferers feel better again. Now they change jobs to more polluted environments and symptoms come back. To offset this, the sufferers put themselves back on the diet that helped before the summer. They get a little better, but now new stresses from the new job cause their immune systems to drop again, so they can't decide if the diet helps or not, so they go off the diet and get even worse!

This is about the time that some doctor tells them "it's all in your head," and they get depressed, so why not try those antidepressants? And these Candida sufferers are depressed, but wouldn't you be? They are depressed because "life" is playing "musical chairs" with their Candida, and they doesn't know it. If they knew what was wrong, they'd be relieved!

Where Does Candida Live?

Candida lives primarily in the gastrointestinal tract. It also lives on or in all the mucus membranes of the body, eyes, ears, nose, throat, vagina, genitals, and the skin. The gastrointestinal tract includes the small intestine (the section of approximately 20 feet of tubing into which the stomach empties) and the colon, or large intestine (a wider 4 - 6 feet of tubing that connects to the end of the small intestines and to the rectum). The gastrointestinal tract is a 25 to 35 foot long hose that runs from your mouth to the anus.

Many people consider that the gastrointestinal -- or digestive -- tract is technically outside of your body. That is an interesting viewpoint that holds that the digestive tract can be viewed as a tunnel or cave that runs through a mountain. The true inside of the body is viewed as the areas that contain organs and glands like the liver, heart, lungs, blood vessels, and the like. The intestinal tract is a pathway or conveyor belt that runs through the body that selectively allows only food which fuels or repairs the body to enter. The tract then discards the other materials that it does not need. Food enters the mouth and travels through the tract and eventually comes out the anus. From the rectum, feces are eliminated from the body into your toilet.

Water helps to float foods through the digestive tract. The stream of water helps push foods through. Whenever we eat something, the intake stimulates muscular contractions that are called *peristalsis*. These are wave-live contractions of muscles that help push or squeeze the foods floating in the stream of water through the entire digestive tract. When food enters your mouth and you begin to chew, saliva is produced that mixes with the food. The saliva has an enzyme called *ptyalin*. This is a starch-digesting enzyme that starts to breakdown the foods as soon as they enter our mouths: sugars from fruits, starches from pastas and bread, and so on. The *parotid glands* located behind the ears and jaw then start to release hormones that stimulate the immune system to be on guard for allergens, toxins, and harmful germs like parasites and bacteria. The parotids put a chemical tag on all the substances in the mouth and those tags tell the immune system whether or not the substance is good or bad, whether it should be attacked or treated as a friendly food substance.

The esophagus is the next stop in the digestive process. It takes about six seconds for food to pass through esophagus. Dry food can get stuck there and take minutes to pass. At the bottom of the esophagus is a tiny trap door called the *cardiac* or *esophageal sphincter*. This muscle is supposed close once it allows food to drop through to the stomach. If for one reason or another the esophageal sphincter remains open once food passes through, a mixture of food and stomach acid and food mixtures can spills back up, and we feel "heartburn." This upward spilling of acid and food is called "Gastric Reflux" and can be caused by a hiatal hernia.

The stomach is the next stop in the digestive process. When food enters the stomach, this muscular organ chops, dices, and blends the foods like a mixing machine. The stomach turns the food into a soupy mixture and produces acids that start to break down proteins. A substance called *pepsin* is also released in the stomach and works to further break down the proteins. The acids also kill unfriendly germs and parasites. Mucus protects the lining of your stomach from the acids. The stomach makes something that has been called *intrinsic factor*. It binds to vitamin B12 to help with absorption into your body. Unfortunately, the older we get the less acid and intrinsic factors we make.

After the stomach comes the small intestine. It is between 15 and 20 feet long and has three parts. Different nutrients are absorbed in each part. The small intestine is where food undergoes the final steps in digestion and is then absorbed into the blood. Tiny hair like fingers called "villi" and smaller ones called "microvilli" absorb the vitamins, minerals, fats, proteins, and sugars that have been broken down from our foods.

The lining of the intestinal tract repairs itself every three to five days. If damage occurs to this lining, harmful things can pass through and cause allergies, arthritis, migraines, headaches, and a host of problems. This is now referred to as "Leaky Gut Syndrome."

The intestinal tract has two other small pipelines connected to it.

One is from the gall bladder, which releases a fluid called *bile* into the intestines to help with the digestion of fats. The pancreas also has a pipeline that releases a fluid called *pancreatin* into the intestines. This fluid contains enzymes that help digest all foods.

The colon – or large intestine -- is the last major part of the intestine. It is 3 - 5 feet in length, and its job is to reabsorb water and any remaining nutrients. Two and one half gallons of water pass through the colon every day. The intestinal tract also contains several pounds of bacteria. Not all this bacteria is disease producing; most of it is friendly and beneficial to us. Of the friendly organism, three are the most abundant. Acidophilus, bifidus, and E coli. The E coli bacteria found in the intestinal tract is not harmful, belongs in the tract, and is said to be a *gram-negative* bacteria. The term *gram negative* refers to the group or type of bacteria that have a thinner cell wall with distinct layers. The other two beneficial bacteria – acidophilus and bifidus -- are said to be *gram-positive* bacteria (gram positive have a different chemical structure then gram negative). These bacteria are available in food such as yogurt, buttermilk, miso, kefir, and some other fermented products. Bifidus bacteria are found in mother's milk and are the dominant bacteria in our intestinal tract during infancy. At some point as a child gets older, Acidophilus begins to grow. Bifidus remains the principle bacteria in our colon, while acidophilus is the principle bacteria in the vaginal area and small intestine. Both bifidus and acidophilus create healthy acids in the intestinal tract that many harmful organisms do not like. These acids adjust the pH range of the intestines. (pH stands for "potential of hydrogen," and indicates how much hydrogen can exist in one place.) The pH range indicates how acid or alkaline the environment is. The acids created by bifidus and acidophilus create a pH range in the intestines of 6.0 to 7.2. Bad organisms have trouble living in this range as they prefer a range well over 7.2. In that type of environment, the bad organisms can eat and breathe easier. When the pH drops, bad organisms have trouble breathing and digesting their own food.

Acidophilus and bifidus also use many harmful organisms as food. In particular, bifidus and acidophilus eat Candida. There are harmful bacteria, viruses and parasites passing through the gastrointestinal tract constantly. The friendly organisms we just discussed repel them and fight them off, so they do not harm us. The good organisms help create a surrounding environment that is hostile to these harmful organisms that we think of as our enemies: things like the cold and flu viruses and many of the bacteria and parasites that cause food poisoning. The friendly organism help digest our food. They literally start to eat our food and create chemical changes that make it easier for us to further break down the food. The friendly organisms also produce small amounts of a few important B vitamins for us. They manufacture these vitamins from left overs they find in our intestines.

If anything happens to damage or kill off these friendly bacteria, Candida and parasites will start to grow out of control. The gastrointestinal tract is home to both Candida and the friendly organisms, and Candida serves a useful purpose: It is food for the friendly organisms. Friendly organisms eat Candida and stay healthy themselves. Being healthy, they can then protect and help us. If we had no Candida at all, the friendly organisms could not use it for food and may not be easily nourished.

Imagine the gastrointestinal tract as being a pond. In this pond live a type of friendly fish called that are called acidophilus and that are the predominant fish in our pond. The acidophilus like to eat other fish in the pond. There is another species of fish that can produce large amounts of waste that could make the water really cloudy and dirty: these waste-producing fish are called *Candida*. The acidophilus fish like to eat Candida fish. They eat them routinely and keep the Candida fish population low enough that the water stays clear. However, the acidophilus don't eat the Candida fish to the point of extinction; rather, they leave enough Candida fish for the species to survive and to continue to act as food for the acidophilus fish but not enough to allow the Candida to take over. If something happened to the acidophilus fish in our pond and they began to die off, their population would decrease, and eventually there would not be enough acidophilus to eat enough of the Candida fish to keep the Candida population a minority in the pond. Soon, the Candida fish would be present in much higher numbers than normal.

The increasing number of Candida fish would begin to release so many waste products into the pond that the pond water would become dirty and polluted. This filthy water would be a perfect breeding ground for harmful bacteria, parasites, and other germs. Soon other forms of life like plants, algae, insects, and other fish would begin to die. They only organisms to really thrive in the polluted pond would be the Candida fish and their harmful friends. There would always some other fish and life in the pond, as the fittest of them would survive, but the pond would not the healthy environment it once was.

This is what happens when the friendly organisms die-off and the Candida and bad ones take over. The intestines become dirty and toxic and become a breeding ground for disease and germs. The takeaway from this overview is that it is important to understand that there are good organism and bad ones. Not all bacteria are bad; many are healthy and protect or serve us. Even the bad ones like Candida and parasites can serve a purpose, like being food for good organisms. A balance is what is needed, not complete domination by either the good or the bad.

What Does Candida Eat?

The bad news about Candida is what it eats. Candida loves starches and sugars. Any food that has an abundant amount of starch or sugar is a friend to Candida. It doesn't matter whether the food is from a health food store, from your local supermarket, from a fast food chain, or from the local drug dealer on the corner. It doesn't matter if it's a health food or a junk food. As long as the food is a starch or a sugar, the Candida love it and can live on it.

Candida can eat certain sugars and foods straight from your intestinal tract as the food comes down. It also eats by way of a root system. As Candida grows, it develops a root system that breaks through the intestinal tract looking for food. These roots tap the tiny blood vessels and absorb glucose which is your blood sugar. These are the two ways that Candida eats.

There have been many different theories on what is the proper diet to use if you have been told that you have Candida. Some diets stress organic foods free of preservatives, colorings, and other additives. Other diets stress vegetarianism as has healthful way to regain balance and to detoxify the body. Some have advocated fasting on fruit and vegetables juice. Some say eat carbs while others say don't eat carbs. Some issues can be misleading; for instance, yeasts love iron, it is an essential nutrient for them. However, eating a low iron diet will just make you more anemic because the yeast is already taking your iron. This approach is not a good long term solution. If you were to go online and search for "Candida diets," you'd be left spinning like a top!

There are probably as many opinions on Candida diets as there are strains Candida. I feel that if one has an effective protocol to eliminate Candida, being extreme with the diet to the point of it becoming truly an esoteric diet is not necessary. Low carbohydrate diets are "far out enough." You do not need to leave your home, move into a cave on the side of a mountain in Virginia that is facing away from all known radio magnetic frequency that begin with "C," eat only foods that have been blessed by monks, and pray to the great god of yeast "Yeasto Beasto."

Let's examine the facts.

1. The common popular belief to date is that yeast eats sugars and starches as PRIMARY foods. The group that will feed Candida the easiest are the free and fermented sugars.

   A. Fermented sugars from alcohol, maltose from beer, and lactose from yogurt (yes yogurt! If has sugars that feed yeast!) are predigested sugar for Candida. This is like throwing gasoline on a fire.

   B. Foods such as fruit sugars and "white sugar" from common junk foods are free sugars and also serve Candida well! Any sugar or sweetener that comes in a powder or liquid probably is a free sugar.

   C. Certain concentrated sugars are NOT good foods for Candida. Honey, for instance, is not a sugar that Candida can freely eat. In fact, there is strong evidence that suggests that honey is an antifungal and can fight Candida. Once honey is eaten, digested, and taken into the blood stream to become part of our blood sugar, Candida may eat freely of it.

2. The next group is the complex carbohydrate group. Starches from potatoes, breads, cereals, noodles, and pasta are called complex carbohydrates. The chemical structures of these "sugars" is much more complex than that of free and fermented sugars, and the body must put these foods through more chemical reactions to break them down to simple sugars. These foods serve as slower forms of foods for the Candida to eat. They must be digested and absorbed into the blood stream to become part of our blood sugar before the Candida will feast on them fully.

3. There is no evidence that eating foods that are of the same genus as fungi or yeast cause Candida as they are not Candida. There is no Candida in a mushroom; therefore, eating a mushroom cannot give you Candida. However, when you have Candida, your immune system is constantly reacting to fungal and yeast proteins. After a while it starts to

believe that all fungal and yeast proteins are bad. The process starts to form an equation that goes like this: "I am being attacked by Candida. Candida is a yeast and a fungus, and it is bad. Mushrooms, brewer's yeast, vinegar, and fermented foods all have yeast or fungal proteins in them; therefore, all yeast and fungal proteins are the same as Candida because Candida is a yeast or fungus. They are all bad and I will be allergic to them."

Now I am not saying this is logical, but this is how the body "thinks." The body reacts to foods of this category not necessarily because they feed the Candida, but because the body views them as being similar. I have encountered many Candida patients who could tolerate these foods and many who had violent reactions to them. What needs to be made clear is fungi and yeasts do not feed Candida in the same way as the fermented sugars, free sugars, and complex carbohydrates do. If foods are high in starches or sugars, they will and can feed the Candida. The extra "kick" they have is the allergic reaction your body has to them. Generally, it is best to avoid fungi and yeasts because they can put added strain on your immune system. But understand that they do not cause Candida nor do they excessively feed it!

Food reactions can often be cut short by taking alka-seltzer gold tablets, baking soda, and potassium bicarbonate in water(ask your pharmacist) or Epsom salts in water.

Gluten

Gluten is a protein found to be connected with "Celiac disease" and mouth sores. Twenty-five percent of the people with recurring mouth sores have elevated antibodies to gluten. When these people stop eating gluten, the mouth sores go away. About half the people with celiac are also lactose intolerant. Gluten sensitivity may be caused by "leaky gut syndrome" which can be caused by Candida.

The symptoms of gluten intolerance are **very similar** to Candida symptoms. The following list of symptoms is common to both:

- **Chronic fatigue**
- **Weakness**
- **Dizziness**
- **Headaches**
- **Cold sweats and/or night sweats**
- **Feeling bad all over, like having the flu**
- **Muscle and joint pains**
- **Numbness, especially in the hands or feet** -
- **Asthma**
- **Chronic sinusitis**
- **Allergies**
- **Irritability**
- **Abdominal pain**
- **Constipation or diarrhea**
- **Gas**
- **Feeling worse when deprived of sugar-containing foods or simple carbohydrates such as potatoes**
- **Feeling worse when exposed to mold, dust, chemicals, or pollutants**
- **General reproductive problems**
- **Premenstrual syndrome-like symptoms**
- **Irregular menstrual cycles or unusual menstrual discharge**

It has been observed that the protein found in wheat, oats, barley, and rye called gluten will worsen the symptoms of Candida patients. I CANNOT find any authoritative material that supports the belief that gluten feeds Candida. It seems to be more of a "rumor" then a fact. Many do agree that Candida suffers worsen when they eat gluten.

What Candida Doesn't Eat

Candida has very little use for low carbohydrate foods. These include green vegetables, most salad vegetables, fish, chicken, turkey, meats, eggs, and game meats. It is that simple.

How to Construct a Candida Diet

Theoretically, it is not necessary to eat animal protein on a Candida diet. There is nothing magical about meat that makes Candida "go away." Meat is low in carbs and sugars and therefore does not make a very good food for Candida. When constructing a Candida diet it is very important to ask yourself these four questions:

1. Does this substance I am about to eat or drink contain free sugars or fermented sugars?
2. Is it high in carbohydrates?
3. Does it contain mycotoxins or substances to which I may have an allergic reaction?
4. If I eat this, how many carbs or sugars will I have consumed for the day?

For Candida patients, the magic number for carbohydrates-consumed-in-a-day appears to be a maximum of 120 to 150 grams. There are diets that go lower. The "Induction Diet" of Dr. Atkins allows around 25 grams a day. This may not be necessary for handling Candida.

When following a Candida diet, it is necessary to have a book which contains the carbohydrate totals found in many different foods. You must add up the typical foods you would want to eat in a day based on one of the following three diets and make sure that the amounts of carbs is less than 150 grams. If your Candida program is not going well, you may wish to consider going lower.

The first diet -- The Candida/Yeast Diet – allows between 100 - 150 grams-a-day. The second --The Strict Candida Diet – allows between 75-125 grams of carbs. The third --The Caveman Diet – allows between 25-75 grams of carbs.

The bad news is that no one can tell you how many carb is right for you. All anyone can do is estimate. You have to discover this for yourself by seeing how you feel.

The Good News is that at the end of this book is an easy to follow Candida diet and cookbook.

Chapter 3

The Vitamin & Mineral Connection

In considering the interactions between nutrients and Candida, we have three categories of reaction that are of interest. The first category includes those nutrients that may feed -- and therefore spread -- the Candida infection. The second category includes nutrients that are neutral and so have little to no effect on the Candida organism. The third and final category occurs when a nutrient has a protective action against the Candida organism.

Nutrients that may feed or nourish the Candida organism include the following:

- **Vitamin D** is an ergosterol (an alcohol steroid found in ergot and other fungi), and it that works to strengthen the membrane of the Candida and so reinforces that membrane. The drug ketoconazole works two ways: it effectively blocks Vitamin D, and it blocks Vitamin D uptake by the Candida organism.
- **Copper** could be the the subject of its own book in terms of how it affects Candida. Copper is very estrogenic; that is, it has estrogen-like growth factors and actions in the body and works as an estrogen enhancer. Copper aggravates Candida because the spread of estrogen is stimulating to the Candida .
- **The B complex vitamins** are very important in influencing the growth of Candida. The B complex vitamins have the ability to convert starches and sugars into simpler and easier forms of sugar on which the Candida organism can feed. B complex vitamins when taken in the presence of carbohydrate foods will feed the Candida organism. Individual B vitamins are not so much the issue.
- **Toxic metals** are another story and an interesting issue unto themselves.

- Two potential toxic elements -- **bismuth** and **aluminum** -- have the potential of alkalizing the intestinal tract and, thereby, raise the intestinal pH to over 7.4 which is the environment in which Candida thrives.
- **Arsenic** and **mercury** have been shown to have a suppressive effect on intestinal immune response and intestinal antibodies and so create an environment that allows Candida to grow and spread based on weakened immunity. Candida has been falsely ascribed the ability to protect the human body by absorbing mercury. This fallacy may be attributed to the observation that, often, when Candida is killed large amounts of mercury escape from the Candida cells. The reality is that in the presence of mercury, Candida grows and multiplies. It is utterly illogical to assume that because Candida absorbs mercury the Candida is doing some great favor to the body.
- **Iron** as an element also stimulates the growth of Candida. The antifungal drug nystatin prevents Candida from absorbing iron therefore interfering with its nutrition.
- **Calcium** is also a vital nutrient for Candida and is essential to the metabolism of Candida. In ways which are not fully understood, Coenzyme Q10 has the ability to spread Candida infections.

The group of nutrients which are protective to the Candida organism include any nutrient that qualifies as an antioxidant. Most prescription antifungal drugs and most vital medicines or herbal medicines work by creating oxidative stress on the membrane of the Candida cell. This oxidative stress damages the membrane of the Candida cell and causes the cell to leak therefore damaging it and allowing one's immune system to be able to more easily invade the Candida cell. So, any nutrient deemed to be an antioxidant (examples are beta-carotene, vitamin E, selenium, vitamin C, lipoic acid, and germanium) or which have antioxidant properties, will serve as antidotes to the medicines that try to kill Candida. Patients' attempts to have the most success on the Candida elimination begins with an agreement to take virtually no supplements during their treatment except for the supplements that are recommended by the Biamonte Center, The interactions that are discussed here are valid from theoretical knowledge, from empirical knowledge, and from observations on how various prescription drugs work to damage the Candida organism. Unfortunately, there have not been any studies to prove the theories posed here.

Nutrients with Protective Action Against Candida

- **Magnesium.** This common mineral is essential to energy levels, bone strength, mood, and much more; yet, the majority of us are not getting anywhere near enough magnesium in our diets. Chronic magnesium deficiency leads to a number of different diseases and conditions, and it can worsen the symptoms of Candida too. Magnesium is required for more than 300 essential biochemical reactions in the body including helping us to produce energy, maintain a healthy nervous system, and regulate blood sugar. It also plays a vital role in removing the toxic byproducts of Candida.
- **Magnesium Deficiency Can Worsen Candida Symptoms:** A lack of magnesium can worsen your Candida symptoms for one simple reason: Magnesium is needed to break down the toxic metabolites of Candida Albicans. Without enough magnesium, your body simply is unable to do the job of removing these substances. Molybdenum is another mineral that works with magnesium in eliminating Candida waste products.

The byproducts of Candida Albicans include ethanol, uric acid and ammonia, but the most important is acetaldehyde. Acetaldehyde is a neurotoxin that affects your brain, nervous system, and many other internal organs. Acetaldehyde also damages your red blood cells and reduces the capacity of your blood to carry oxygen around the body. If your body is unable to effectively process and remove Acetaldehyde, this toxic substance can affect many different systems and cause a variety of symptoms. Acetaldehyde is also produced when you drink alcohol, and it is thought to be the primary cause of the next morning's hangover!

Although magnesium is not the only nutrient needed to break down acetaldehyde, it plays a major role. There is one particular enzyme that your body needs to turn toxic acetaldehyde into harmless acetate. Called aldehyde dehydrogenase, it requires magnesium to function properly. Without enough magnesium, your body is unable to activate the aldehyde dehydrogenase, which is therefore unable to break down acetaldehyde, which in turn can lead to symptoms like headaches and fatigue.

Candida Causes Magnesium Deficiency, Too

I just explained how a lack of magnesium can make Candida symptoms worse, but you should know that Candida can also prevent you from getting enough magnesium in the first place. Health issues are rarely a case simply of one thing leading to another, and this is a great example of how cause and effect are often inextricably linked. In this case, Candida Albicans actually prevents you from getting enough of the very mineral you need to combat its effects. This is why Candida sufferers are often even more deficient in magnesium.

In the early stages of a Candida overgrowth, your body copes relatively well with the extra waste products that need to be eliminated. Your liver and kidneys are working effectively, your digestive system is functioning well and your body's various elimination pathways are doing what they should. The acetaldehyde, uric acid, and other Candida metabolites are being efficiently removed. However, as your gut flora becomes more compromised and the yeast-bacteria imbalance starts to grow, your body starts to become overwhelmed.

As increasing amounts of the Candida metabolites begin to appear, more and more of your magnesium is used to break them down. If you started with a healthy surplus of magnesium, it might take some time for you to become deficient. If you were deficient already (like most of us), then the onset of the typical Candida symptoms might happen very quickly. Without changes in diet or supplementation, your body simply runs out of the nutrients that it needs to process these toxins. As if that weren't enough, we also need to factor in the effect that Candida has on your digestion. When the balance of gut flora in your small intestine is compromised, your gut loses much of its ability to extract and absorb nutrients from your food. A primary role of the small intestine is to absorb the micronutrients that you eat in your food. When it is unable to perform this role adequately, you can become deficient in many of the vitamins and minerals (including magnesium) that you need to recover your health.

So, as you can see, the development of a Candida overgrowth can lead to magnesium deficiency in two ways. First, it depletes the (probably limited) stores of magnesium that you already have. And secondly, it interferes with your body's ability to absorb more magnesium from your diet. Add in the fact that most of us have barely enough magnesium to start with, and it becomes apparent how easily the Candida yeast can benefit from a lack of this important mineral.

Testing for Magnesium

A hair mineral analysis is a very good test to measure to tissue levels of magnesium. The average level will be between 3 and 6 milligrams percent. Levels above 6.9 milligrams percent do not indicate an excess, but rather a loss out of the body. Just as steam can escape from a kettle, so can magnesium and other minerals leach out of our cells. These minerals can then be found in excess in our hair and other tissues.

Why are we deficient in magnesium? The answer lies in the way that our diets have changed.

The first culprit is modern-day farming practices. Although intensive farming has been around for less than 100 years, that has been sufficient time to strip farmed soil of many of its nutrients. Studies have shown that the magnesium levels in today's vegetables are at least 25 percent lower than they were before 1950. Depleted soil leads to less nutritious food, which contributes to lower magnesium levels in your blood and tissues.

Meanwhile, the way that your food is processed has a huge effect on its magnesium content as well. According to some sources, refined pastas and breads contain 80 – 95 percent less magnesium than the whole grain equivalent. If you needed another reason to avoid refined grains (and there are plenty of reasons!), there it is.

The content of our diets is different now too. We eat more refined grains, fewer vegetables, and fewer nuts and seeds. In other words, we eat more of the foods that contain little magnesium and much less of the foods that are rich in it. This has become such a problem that many people in developed countries get a large part of their magnesium from foods like French fries and beer -- simply because those are the foods that they consume the most!

Finally, the diabetes and obesity epidemics that are sweeping the world might also be playing a role in magnesium deficiency. There is a close relationship between low magnesium levels and high blood sugar. Just as a high sugar diet can contribute to a magnesium deficiency, so a lack of magnesium seems to disrupt blood sugar regulation.

Does Magnesium promote Candida?

There are some who will tell you that magnesium 'feeds' or stimulates Candida in some way or promotes the formation of *biofilms*. There is some truth in this, in that Candida does actually need magnesium to survive. But then so do all living organisms! Restricting your magnesium intake to combat Candida thereby deliberately making yourself magnesium-deficient would be about as effective as trying to breath less oxygen. On the other hand, eliminating sources of excess sugar (like the Candida Diet does) is a much more practical and effective goal.

- **Taurine, Choline and Vitamin B6**
  These are very important co-factors of helpers of magnesium. If a patient is taking magnesium and the symptoms of magnesium deficiency do not go away, or if magnesium levels do not improve on a test, very often the person needs to add these co-factors. Vitamin B6 helps the absorption and utilization of magnesium. Choline and magnesium help regulate fats, cholesterol, and other lipids. Taurine and magnesium help regulate the heart beat and keep the heart from beating irregularly or skipping beats.

Other Vitamins & Minerals

Candida Promoters: (Promote Growth / Inhibit Immune Response)

- **Co Enzyme Q10** – Increases energy production in Candida
- **Vitamin D** – Improves membrane function in Candida. Many anti-fungal drugs work by inhibiting Candida's ability to utilize Vitamin D.
- **B Complex** – Allows your body to convert sugars into fuel for Candida.
- **Excess Iron** – Feeds Candida growth

- **Excess Copper** – Lowers adrenal and immune function, allowing Candida to grow.
- **Excess Antioxidants** – Certain anti-fungal treatments work to kill Candida by using free radicals. If these free radicals are quenched, these therapies may be less effective.

Candida Neutral (seem to have no effect):

- **Fish Oils** (EPA & DHA)
- **Vitamin E**
- **Bioflavonoids**
- **Molybdenum** – helps to detoxify by-products of "Die Off"

Candida Inhibiters:

- **Selenium** – Boosts immunity
- **Vitamin C** – Boosts immunity (Don't use with Manganese & copper deficient patients)

Chapter 4

The Biamonte Method – An Overview

The Biamonte Method of Candida Elimination is divided into five separate sections – or phases. Besides having its own unique mechanism in eliminating Candida, each phase is also designed to prepare the body for the phase that follows. This ensures that each phase will work correctly. As an example, the second phase will not work correctly if the first phase was not done to full completion and so on.

The reason for the five sections is that is has been found that Candida must be eliminated or stripped out of the body in "layers." This is due to Candida having different stages of growth were it will exist in different forms. Like a chameleon, Candida is able to transform itself from a fungus into yeast. I firmly believe that using an approach that attempts to correct all of the patient's imbalances, symptoms, or deficiencies simultaneously will aggravate the Candida. Certain vitamins, minerals, amino acids, and herbs can spread Candida while others protect it from the very medicines used to kill it.

The Biamonte method addressed early on two situations that have a major impact on Candida: these are toxic metals and hormone imbalances. Both have been found to be underlying causes of Candida. However, it is how they are addressed not the mere fact that they are addressed that makes the difference between success and failure.

An Outline of the Five Phases of Candida Elimination

Phase 0

Many years ago, I discovered that parasites could cause Candida. This is covered in other articles and writings that you can find on our web site. The exact mechanics of this is simple. Parasites destroy friendly flora just like antibiotics do. Many parasites excrete ammonia and other toxic chemicals that destroy friendly flora like acidophilus. Some parasites also depress the immune response in the intestinal tract allowing yeasts to overgrow. Anything that destroys friendly flora can cause an overgrowth of Candida since friendly flora holds Candida in check.

The purpose of Phase 0 is to eliminate enough of the parasites from the lining of the intestinal tract so that the person will not quickly relapse on Phase 1. Phase 0 also eliminates the top layers of Candida growth so there is less die-off from Phase 1 that could make you feel sick. This also allows Phase 1 to absorb faster and deeper into your system.

Phase 1

The purpose of Phase 1 is to eliminate and destroy most of the Candida in the body. This program destroys Candida in the intestines, the blood, lymph and vital organs.

This is known as the *rotation program*. Once we have tested the person to discover the type of Candida they have, we select four substances that are especially effective on that type of Candida. The first chosen substance is taken for a 4-day period and then stopped. Then the second substance is taken for the next 4 day; the third for four days, and the fourth for another 4 days. The process is repeated over and over again. The rotation is done so that the Candida does not develop a resistance to any of the substances. (This concept is covered in my earlier articles on Candida)

At this time hormones are checked and a program to correct them is begun as an adjunct. If the hormones are imbalanced, the Candida will not fully clear, and Phase 1 will not kill all of its intended victims!

Phase 2

Phase 2 has three purposes:

1) To destroy the Candida buried in the intestinal tract. If this Candida is not removed it will eventually cause a full-blown relapse within six months to year.
2) To establish friendly bacteria in the intestinal tract and to stimulate the immune response in the intestines' that fights Candida and harmful organisms. This is not done in Phase 1 or Phase 0 because we have proved that Candida will prevent friendly acidophilus and bifidus bacteria from growing. The Candida must be eliminated before the friendly bacteria will grow. An analogy would be trying to plant flowers in a garden of weeds.
3) To repair any damage to the intestines tract (leaky gut) that has occurred and that may be causing food allergies and chemical sensitivities. At this time, the fecal toxic metal test is performed to check for the metals referred to in the "Toxic Metal Connection" mentioned earlier in this article.

Phase 3

The purpose of Phase 3 is to completely eliminate all toxic metals and then to correct any deficiency of vitamins, minerals, amino acids, hormones, or fatty acids that exists. Special tests are performed to measure all the nutrients. The most common mistake in trying to regain energy patients who have Candidiasis is the use of many vitamins and minerals or other exotic supplements intended to boost energy while the Candida still exists in the body.

Giving a toxic body dozens of nutrients is to ask for trouble. People can become severely ill if they take many nutrients when they are chronically toxic. The nutrients will cause a mad, uncontrolled release of toxins which the body was not prepared to release. The result will be feeling terrible. Candida sufferers usually get bad reactions to vitamin supplements. This is why vitamins are not given until Phase 3, after the

Candida is gone.

Phase 4

The purpose here is to stimulate the immune system. In order to prevent relapse of Candida or any chronic viral condition, proper immune function must be restored. After Phase I and Phase 2 (killing the yeast) and Phase 3 (restoring vitamin and mineral balance and energy) have been completed, the immune system is perfectly set up to be restored. Immune function will not come back if we have deficiencies and toxic metals as these problems can suppress the immune system. You certainly cannot restore the immune system while you have an active Candida infection. If your house were on fire (which is like having an infection), would you put out the fire or would you run into the burning house with new rugs, wallpaper, and furniture and try to "build the house back up" while it was burning down? Special testing may be done to measure immune function.

Why The Five Phase Biamonte Method Work!

The Biamonte Method has a success rate of better than 90 percent according to our recent surveys. Much of the success of this approach is not in *what* we do, but in *when* we do it and in what we *DO NOT DO*!

Mixing these phases together would result in patients who either respond slowly, do not respond at all, or who get worse. Most doctors get poor results with Candida because they fail to understand the interactions between Candida, vitamins, hormones, and toxic metals

The true benefit and importance of this program is in preventing relapse. This program is has two basic purposes: to eliminate Candida using our advanced methods and to prevent Candida relapse by systematically correcting all the know causes.

Chapter 5

The Biamonte Method of Testing: An Interview

Interviewer: *Doctor, can you tell us more about the Biamonte Method of Testing?*

Dr Biamonte: The urine is tested within the first hour of voiding for accuracy. After the hour has passed, chemical reactions will occur that will lower the accuracy.

The Candida test measures chemical waste products from harmful bacteria and parasites, waste products that are produced as a by-product of Candida's own metabolisms, and free radical reactions that occur from the alcohol by-products of Candida. Bacteria. Yeasts and parasites produce "organic acids" unique to themselves. This can be thought of as chemicals that are produced by the organisms that are not produced by our own bodies. These chemicals serve as "footprints" of these organisms.

We measure these wastes in the urine to determine if they are in a range we consider to be consistent with Candida overgrowth. Those who have a poor immune system can experience "Candida symptoms" at low levels. When we kill these organisms, the organic acids or waste products will increase. This is because the organism is dying, decomposing, and releasing these chemicals. The first Candida test that we do serves as a baseline.

The very first urine test we suggest to a new client is performed as a "Challenge" or "Provocation" test. This typically is done when testing for toxic chemicals or toxic metals levels in the body.

We have the client do a baseline , and they then enter Phase 0 of our program for 3 - 4 weeks. Phase 0 is intended to mechanically remove and dislodge Candida, bacteria, and parasites from the intestinal lining. The client then repeats the urine test to ascertain changes that occur between the first test and the second as a result of the loosening and scrubbing action.

The second urine test will often reveal organisms that may have been brought out of hiding. Sometimes levels increase on the second test indicating that Candida was hiding in the intestines and not reacting with the person's immune response.

In other cases Candida levels may drop, but the parasite levels may rise indicating that Candida is not the primary infection but that parasites are. Sometimes the Candida levels remain high, and the results of the first and second tests indicate they are unaffected by the Phase 0. This indicates that there are colonies of Candida that have moved outside of the intestinal tract and have invaded other parts of the body. These colonies were not affected by the intestinal cleansing of Phase 0 so the levels remain unchanged.

When the client begins the Candida program, we expect the organic acid levels to go higher as a result of the program killing the organisms. At some point they will start to drop. This signals that the phase we are on is reaching its end and that the current regimen has reached and killed all the Candida it is able to kill. This is a signal that the next phase should begin. After starting the next phase, the new substance begins to attack the Candida in a new area or location of the body. This causes the level of Candida organic acids to rise again. At some point they will drop, again signaling the end of that phase.

When we have used the final group of substances that are used to destroy the Candida in the intestinal membrane and we have achieved a drop in the organic acid level, we can assume the overgrowth of

Candida is eliminated, and it is now time to concentrate on building up the levels of friendly bacteria to take its place.

The Biamonte Method of testing represents the first test for Candida that is designed to complement a Candida elimination program. The method reports the level of die-off the program is producing. Unlike other methods, if the client feels worse on the program as a result of the dead Candida, the test will reflect that so we can understand whether or not the "feeling worse" is a result of the program killing the Candida or the person feeling bad for some other reason. This is a time when consultation with the regular medical doctor treating the client may be considered to opinion that doctor's thoughts regarding the reason.

In the past, our Candida testing also employed an advanced stool culture called the Chromagar. The Chromagar test identifies the species of Candida in the body of the client. This was used because I have found that certain substances or herbs will work better on certain types or strains of Candida. However after years and years of refining our protocols, we no longer need the stool test information. At this time, the substances that we use in our protocol are able to destroy all organisms. We may add the stool test in some cases, but it is generally not needed any longer.

Chapter 6

Phase 0:
An Interview

Interviewer: *Can you describe Phase 0 of the Biamonte Method along with the supplements you recommend?*

Dr Biamonte: Phase 0 is our starting point to eliminate Candida. Without Phase 0, patients can get strong herxhiemer reactions from the phases 1 and 2 which are the most aggressive of the program.

Many years ago I discovered that parasites may play a role in the promotion of Candidal overgrowth. This is covered in other articles and writings that you can find on our Web site, www.Health-Truth.com. The mechanics of this is simple. Like antibiotics, parasites destroy healthy flora. They do this by excreting ammonia and other toxic chemicals that destroy healthy bacteria like Lactobacillus and Acidophilus. Some parasites also depress the immune response in the intestinal tract allowing Candida to overgrow. Anything that destroys friendly flora can cause an overgrowth of Candida since friendly flora holds Candida in check.

Constipation can also cause Candida, by causing the bowel pH to become far too alkaline and encourage the growth of parasites. Candida likes a slow moving, toxic bowel. The intention of Phase 0 is both to correct -- or prevent-- constipation and to eliminate some of the parasites/ Candida living on the surface of the intestinal tract. Notice I say some!

Phase 0 will not remove it all, nor is it intended to do so. Its purpose is to remove enough of the organisms during a one month period to allow the following phases to cause less reaction and to work faster.

Another purpose of Phase 0 is to eliminate enough of the parasites from the lining of the intestinal tract so that the person will not quickly relapse on Phase 1. Phase 0 also eliminates the top layers of Candida growth, so there is less die-off from Phase 1 that could make you feel sick. This also allows the Phase 1 rotation to absorb faster and deeper into your system. There are generally three supplements used on Phase 0, although others could be used depending on the patient's case.

The Loosener
One of the supplements used in Phase 0 chemically loosens the Candida and parasites off the walls of the intestinal tract. This product contains substances that break the "glue like" bonds that the organisms use to attach or adhere to the intestinal lining. The ingredients in this product also help to heal "leaky gut" to a minor degree. As long as there is significant Candida growth in the intestines, the leaky gut will not be able to heal. However this product can heal it enough to help cut back some of the reactions that the patient may have to foods, chemicals, and to the products that eliminate the Candida.

The Scraper
This formula scraps off the top layer of Candida by tearing into the outside membrane as if the Candida were being attacked by thousands of tiny knives. It contains Diatomaceous (die-a-toe-may-shus) Earth which consists of the pulverized sea shells from creatures known as diatomes that lived long ago and died in groups so massive that they can, today, be mined and bulldozed.

"DE", as it's abbreviated, has the neat quality of killing insects. (Unfortunately, it kills good ones, like bees and ladybugs, too, so its use shouldn't be indiscriminately.) DE is 100 percent ecologically safe to the environment and non-poisonous to man and beast. In fact, if you've eaten anything made with flour (like Bisquick), you've eaten DE. DE is a great remover of parasites and intestinal yeasts and works by slicing open the exoskeleton (outer, hard covering) of insects, causing them to "bleed" to death. (Actually, their insides leak out, so they dehydrate and die.) This same things happens to yeasts and parasites

When DE is sprinkled on the ground, on an ant mound, or mix it with grains, legumes, or other food products, the DE slices and dices the insects that walk through the product, but DE won't hurt YOU when you ingest it because the 'sharp pieces' are too small to cut you as your membranes are too thick for it to penetrate. (Many farmers deliberately mix DE with animal feed to kill internal parasites in farm animals. The DE in the animal feces even kills the fly maggots that invariably appear in the patties.)

The Sponge

The last of the three formulas used in Phase 0 is used to absorb the loosened Candida and parasites and to carry them out of the body. This formula contains six key ingredients that absorb the organisms much like a sponge and carry them out of the intestinal tract. The product can be used in higher doses as a mild laxative or cleanser. It helps to remove the decaying wastes of parasites and yeasts so that they do not cause toxic reactions.

Because the Phase 0 products do not attack Candida chemically, they do not need to be rotated. Only substances that chemically kill Candida can become ineffective due to an immunity developing. Substances that work mechanically continue to work. If you were trying to poison someone, their body could develop an immunity to the poison, but if you then started to beat them over the head with a bat, they would not develop and immunity to the bat.

Phase 0 is not expected to produce a symptomatic improvement in the patient, though many people report improvements. However, we do not expect any noticeable change except for the bowels moving a bit more. The Phase 0 protocol continues throughout the Phase 1 rotation and into the Phase 2 Intestinal Candida Elimination program.

We have found that it takes no less than six months to eliminate Candida and, in some cases, up to one year. This is because Candida grows deep into the intestinal tract like mold grows into cheese or bread. Regardless of how strong the medicine is, it takes time for the medicine to absorb deeper and deeper into the tissues. This is why medical drugs are not a workable solution for Candida elimination. They are too toxic to be taken for the length of time necessary to eliminate the Candida.

This is why the Phase 0 program is continued throughout Phase 1 and Phase 2: we need to be constantly scrubbing off the next layer of Candida that comes to the surface as old layers of skin die and are thrown off. The new layer growing beneath will reveal the next layer of Candida.

Phase 0 sometimes can eliminate mild cases of parasites and Candida without further protocols. It can be used as a general bowel cleanse as well. But, the most important function of Phase 0 is as your first step in eliminating your Candida.

Interviewer: *Dr Biamonte, I heard that some of your patients are very sensitive to ANY anti-Candidal intervention. Is this true, and how would you approach these easily sensitized patients?*

Dr Biamonte: Yes, some patients can't even tolerate the three formulas used in Phase 0, so in that case I recommend Mucins. They are naturally produced in the intestinal tract of all mammals. They have the same effect as the wax we use on our floors or cars. They protect the intestinal cells from allergens and from reacting to our own friendly flora. Whether it's the eyes, sinuses, throat, chest, or intestinal tract, mucin (from colixen) provides a first line of defense. Mucin is a protein that forms a protective gel layer over all mucous membranes of the body. In the intestinal tract, mucins protect the intestinal lining from the hostile environment of bacteria, viruses, and toxins. Often, when someone reacts very adversely to all supplements and foods, they need to take Mucins for several weeks before attempting the Phase 0 program. In most cases, the use of Mucins allows the person to tolerate the program. In rare cases, an actual leaky gut protocol most be used to heal up the gut to some degree before starting or getting back on Phase 0. We only expect the leaky gut program to improve the patient to the point where the program can continue. Then, when the Candida is eliminated, the leaky gut program is implemented in full as the last step of Phase 2.

[illegible]

Chapter 7

Phase 1: An Interview

Interviewer: *Now that your patients have loosened and removed the top layer of Candida in Phase 0 of your program, where do they go from here?*

Dr Biamonte: In Phase I, our main objective is to eliminate most of the infection in the body, whether it's a virus, bacteria, yeast, fungus, or a parasite.

Phase 1 of the program is a systemic phase. As far as the infection goes, we're trying to eliminate most of the infection throughout most of the body. The things that you're taking on Phase I on your rotation are specific natural and herbal substances that have the ability to be absorbed throughout your blood, to travel through your bloodstream and lymphatic system, and to be able to kill or eliminate most of the infection throughout most of the body.

In Phase I, all of the items that you're taking are rotated. By rotated we mean you'll be switching from one to the next. You're not taking all of these items on the same day; you're taking each item by itself alone for four days. After that four-day period of taking one specific formula, you stop it, and then go to the next item written on your program sheet labeled with a #2. After four days of taking the second formula, you then stop and go to the product labeled #3. And after four days of taking that formula, you then stop that and go to the formula labeled #4. And you keep doing this until you've used all the formulas, whether there are four, five ,or six that you are rotating. After you've finished them all, you go back to the first one again.

We call this a *rotation*, and we call each one of the substances *a rotated formula*, because you're only taking it for four days and then switching to another one.

We expect each one of the formulas to produce some kind of a change in your body, or in how you feel. We're not necessarily expecting you to feel better throughout this entire phase or when you start doing the phase, and we're not exactly expecting you to feel worse either. We're expecting some kind of change. How a change will occur is by the products you're taking. These changes and symptoms are related to the killing of the harmful organisms, viruses, bacteria, yeast, and parasites in your system. As a by-product of these changes, you may have symptoms like gas, headaches, and nausea. Various pains in your joints may occur. A full list of symptoms are on the sheet at the back of the book labeled, "What to Expect on Phase I."

If you feel noticeably better, it's because your body is able to kill the infection and eliminate the dead waste or debris from the infection; and, therefore, you're feeling better. If you feel worse, it's simply because your body cannot fully and quickly eliminate the dead debris from the infection, and this dead waste -- or toxic junk -- is causing your body to feel sick. This is why one person may do the same exact program as another and one may feel bad while the other may feel better. Both of them are getting results, but the person who is feeling better has a body that is better able to eliminate the dead germs that are building up in the system, so the patient is feeling the benefit of killing them and then eliminating them. The other person is definitely killing these germs and getting an improvement in that way, but this patient is not feeling improvement because the dead germs are building up in the system, and the body can't throw them out fast enough. So this patient's body is overwhelmed or toxic. And this is what we mean by a change. You will feel either better or worse.

A "no-change rotated formula" (produces no effect -- you're not feeling better or worse after the month is over) is a formula that has not been efficient or effective on your program and may eventually need to be eliminated and substituted. We can only tell if the formula is a "no-change" after about three to four weeks on your program because at any point in the first thirty days of the program, you may suddenly feel better or worse from a formula that produced no change the first time you took it.

Generally speaking, on the rotation, capsules or tablets are taken with meals. Any liquid is taken on an empty stomach. The ideal would be to take the liquid an hour before you eat or three hours after you eat. The only item that needs to be taken with food on your program is Biocidin or Bioradiance (either one of them should be taken with food to avoid the possibility of intestinal upset). Start at a low dose with your normal-sized meals, and then gradually raise the dose as you find that you're tolerating it. If at any point you don't feel that you're tolerating it, either eat a larger meal or lower the dose of the Biocidin or Bioradiance. These are powerful herbal remedies: so strong that you have to take them with their accompanying product, Biotonic.

Interviewer: *Are there any Phase 1 reactions that patients might experience?*

Dr Biamonte: If you're on Phase I and you're experiencing flu-like symptoms, chances are you are not getting a cold or flu. You are simply getting a die-off reaction. A "die-off" reaction occurs when the germs in your system are being killed off, and their little bodies -- if you want to look at it this way -- are breaking open and releasing their toxins. If you are getting this die-off reaction, the best thing to do is to lower the dose of the remedies that you're taking. By "lowering the dose" we mean to cut it back to whatever dose it takes for you to feel comfortable on that supplement. So, if you're taking half a dropper of something four times a day and getting bad reactions, cut it to half a dropper twice a day. If you're still getting bad reactions, then cut it down to a half a dropper once a day. And if you're still getting bad reactions, cut it down to a quarter of a dropper a day.

What's happening when you get a bad reaction is that these organisms are being killed faster than your body can eliminate them, so you feel sick. When you lower the dose, you're cutting back the speed at which these things are being killed and poisoning your system, so your body is then able to deal with eliminating the dead material at a speed it's comfortable with so you don't feel so bad. You can lower the dose literally to ANY dose going down to an amount that fits on the head of a pin if necessary, in order to feel comfortable.

Also, drinking a lot of distilled water is very helpful. Drinking maybe four ounces of distilled water every half hour is very useful in cutting back the symptoms of the die-off.

Another thing that is very helpful is to take an enema, or to go for a colonic, or use a colema board. An enema is a very low-level approach; the colema and the colonic are much more thorough and allow much more water to pass into the system and clean you out. So, a colema, colonic, or enema will help to flush dead debris out of your intestinal tract or colon, which will make you feel better while you're getting the die-off reaction.

So, the three ways to help cut back on die-off are: 1) lower the dose of what you're taking; 2) drink distilled water, 4 oz every half hour; 3) to take an enema, colema, or colonic.

Phase 1 of the program usually lasts thirty days, and after that you will test your urine and meet with the nutritionist to understand what's happened during the Phase 1 and how well you've done. It's very possible that after the thirty-day period, you might be finished with this phase and move to the Phase 2. It's also possible that you might need to continue the Phase 1 a little longer and perhaps change something in the program. Your nutritionist will know by testing your urine and by asking you the various questions that are on a pre-made form at the back of this book.

Your urine analysis looks for three things. The first is pH, because it tells us the susceptibility or likelihood of you having active infections. The average pH should be at about 6.4, and as it drops to 5 or to below 4, it means the person is more susceptible to having infections living in their body. As the pH goes higher, to 6, 6.5, or even 7, that shows the person is not susceptible to infections, and the infections might have cleared out of the body.

Secondly, we look at is something called *indican*. It's a measurement of the amount of toxicity in your colon and intestines. Indican is produced by food that is putrefying in your intestines, mixing with harmful bacteria, parasites, or yeast, which is then releasing a harmful substance called *indole*. Indole is absorbed into your blood, and the body then eliminates the indole through your urine as a different substance which is called indican. Indican is what we're measuring in your urine.

The last thing we look for in your urine is a protein waste product that is given off by parasites and yeast. Measuring all three of these, along with asking you the different questions, will help us determine whether or not your program is complete, whether you need to continue the phase longer, whether you need to continue the phase and change something in the program, or whether you need to go to the second phase,

The next group of supplements I want to discuss are the supplements that are indicated on your program as "daily supplements." They may include enzymes to help your digestion or to help the rotated items work better. They may also include a specific type of anti-viral, anti-bacterial, anti-parasitic, or anti-yeast agent that needs to be taken every day to boost the speed of the killing or elimination of these organisms. You may also have another substance on your program which might help with elimination. It is very common that people become constipated on Phase I. Constipation on this phase is basically a trouble spot. If you become constipated, you will get an increase in bad reactions. You will get more unpleasant reactions on this phase if you're constipated than if your bowels are moving well. So, your daily item on your program might be something to aid your elimination.

It's also possible that, due to a specific situation or problem that you have, you might be put on a daily supplement of some type to help with some type of chronic complaint that we want to begin addressing right now in Phase I. Generally speaking, taking anti-oxidants which would be beta carotene or Vitamin E, Vitamin C, selenium or zinc, quercetin, pycnogenol, or some other types of vitamins is not a good idea on Phase I. These anti-oxidants could stop some of your rotated items from being able to kill the organisms. If you're on a Candida program, calcium, Vitamin D, and copper are nutrients which can all help support Candida and keep it strong, thereby avoiding being killed by our rotated items. Any person on a Candida program should NOT be taking B-complex vitamins. You may be able to take a singular B vitamin for a specific purpose but taking a B-complex is not a good idea because it also helps the yeast in its own metabolism.

If you're on an anti-viral program, anti-oxidants may also not be a good idea, as we discussed above. Also, on anti-viral programs, calcium, Vitamin D, and copper are nutrients that can stimulate the virus, reactivate it, or keep it in activation. Certain Chinese herbs may also do that. So you should be careful of what you take. Always check with your nutritionist before you add anything to your program.

If you're on an anti-parasitic program, the same would hold true as an anti-Candida program, where the anti-oxidants may be interfering with the ability to kill the parasites. So it is always best that you check with your nutritionist before you take anything.

There are two versions of the Candida Diet on Phase I. One version we call the *Basic List*, which is a basic Candida diet. That's in the back of this book. It's the diet that's generally good for most cases of Candida. It can also be used by vegetarians with minor modifications. It's a little bit more difficult for vegetarians to eliminate Candida if they stay on a vegetarian diet because that diet will tend to be higher in carbohydrates than will the diet of someone else eating meat. We are not endorsing a meat-eating diet as a general health-promoting diet for everybody; we're simply pointing out that on the Candida diet, following a low-carbohydrate diet will help eliminate parasites or Candida as fast as possible. No one is claiming that this is a diet that should be followed by everyone all the time as a health-promoting diet.

Also in the back of this book is the second version of the Candida Diet, the *Caveman Diet* (Better known as Paleo). It's the strictest Candida diet for those who have the toughest cases. That diet is mainly animal protein which includes fish, chicken, all types of red meat, and low carbohydrate vegetables. It's a very simple diet, and that's all there is to it.

Interviewer: *Dr. Biamonte, could you give a quick summary of Phase One?*

Dr Biamonte:

1. The Formulas on your program are rotated and are called rotated Formulas.
2. They're done for four days each, then you stop and move to the next item.
3. The liquids are taken on an empty stomach; all the tablets or capsules are taken with meals.

4. Biocidin and Bioradiance especially must be taken with food; otherwise you may feel intestinal distress and nausea.
5. Formulas that produce no change on your program are referred to as "no-change rotated item Formulas."
6. The program will usually last about 30 days, and then you'll come back into the office with a urine sample to be re-tested–either to go on to Phase 2, or have your program altered or updated in some way.
7. Daily items might be used on your program for specific purposes which will be very individual to you, possibly to assist in better digestion or better elimination through your bowels.
8. We do not expect to eliminate ALL of the infection in the person in this phase.
9. We do not expect ALL the symptoms to go away, or for the person to feel he's totally 100 percent in this phase. That's what the other phases are for.
10. We do expect the severe symptoms of active infection to be eliminated by this phase.
11. It is very important that once you finish Phase I you move immediately to Phase 2.

(PLEASE NOTE: The contents of this chapter are for informational purposes only. It is highly recommended that this program be conducted under the supervision of a qualified healthcare professional educated and certified in the Biamonte Method.)

Chapter 8

Phase 2: An Interview

Interviewer: *So.... Doctor, what happens in Phase 2?*

Dr Biamonte: The goal of Phase 2 is to cleanse the body. By *cleanse* we mean to eliminate any harmful toxins, whether they come from your environment (home, job, air, or water supply) or are produced by your body during its own normal functioning(digestion, exercise, Etc.)

Phase 2 is very important, because Phase 2 is the part of the program where we ensure that we're eliminating all of the infection the system is carrying. In the case of parasites or Candida, these organisms are eliminated on Phase 2 by cleansing the bowel. In the case of viral conditions like Epstein-Barr or cytomeglio virus or other Herpes-type viruses that are associated with chronic fatigue, we eliminate the virus by also cleansing the intestines and by cleaning the liver, the lymphatic system, the spleen, and various other organs and glands that are known to house these viruses. Harmful bacteria are also eliminated on Phase 2 in a similar manner.

In dealing with Candida and parasites, the Phase 2 program will have three steps (for some, it will be reduced to two steps). The first step, Part A, uses four different classifications of supplements. The first group of supplements are classified as "looseners." We call them *looseners* because their job is to loosen old debris -- old mucus or fecal matter -- which is sitting in the intestinal tract and that Candida or parasites or harmful bacteria might be hiding in or buried in. We want to loosen these substances so that we can remove them substance from your system, thereby creating more surface area for good flora to colonize on the intestinal wall. Phase 2, Part A "Looseners" can include castor oil, garlic oil, bromelin, or pancreatin. Pepsin (which is an enzyme produced in your stomach) and comfrey (an herb) also could be used to help eliminate the mucus debris which is stuck in your intestinal tract.

The next formulas that we'll talk about are essentially what we've categorized as the "bulldozer" group. Their job is to come through the intestinal tract and push out old debris that the looseners have loosened. The bulldozer group usually consists of some kind of fiber product, which commonly contains psyllium and benzonite. Psyllium is a fiber that absorbs water and swells up, and benzonite is a clay which is highly absorbent: able to hold many, many poisons and toxins. It can hold several times its weight in toxins and toxic material. The type of fiber products we use to bulldozer out the old material in the bowel are usually in themselves products which contain various herbs which help to purge the intestinal tract of worms or kill parasites and yeast.

The third group of formulas used in this Phase 2, Part A are specific digestive aids. These are things to rebuild the digestive system or to help the digestive system. These can include plant enzymes, hydrochloric acid, pancreatin, or bile salts. These are all things that the body needs and, for the most part, produces on its own in order to digest your food.

The fourth and final group of supplements which might be used are the Candida killers, and these particular killers we categorize as "mop-up" formulas. The reason we call them "mop-up" is because their job is to mop up any remaining Candida from your system and to eliminate it. These mop-up items are a classification of natural anti-fungal substances which, due to the fact that they are essentially an oily type of product, can line your intentional tract just like you were pouring oil down a tube or pipe. They reach yeast that we ordinarily could not reach with other products. Products that absorb into your blood and travel throughout the body killing yeast may not be able to reach the crevices or nooks and crannies that these items can reach.

There's a fifth optional group of supplements which many times is used on people, and these are *vermifuges*. Vermifuges are things that kill vermin, and vermin are worms or parasites. It's pretty much known and accepted through our research that almost everyone with Candida has worms or parasites to a greater or lesser degree. Therefore, it's quite common on Phase 2, Part A, that we have a built-in group of supplements which are given to act as vermifuges to kill and expel any worms or parasites the person might have. Common ones are K-min, black walnut, and butternut bark. These are the three most commonly used because they're the most general, all-purpose ones that work well on just about everyone.

These items are taken all together, with one exception. The Candida killering "mop-up items" are rotated. It's very common on your Phase 2 program that you will have two mop-up items, both rotated four days each, while you're taking all the rest of the supplements every day.

The bulldozer products, the fiber products that clean the intestines, are generally taken on an empty stomach, but only twice a day. It could be that you're taking them three times, but twice is pretty common. The digestive aids are always taken at meals. Any plant enzymes, hydrochloric acid, bile salts, or pancreatin would be taken at meal time. This is to help you digest your food.

The mop-up items, the Candida killers, would also be taken at meal times. The additional items that would purge parasites -- the vermifuge supplements -- could be taken on an empty stomach; but depending on which ones they are, may also be taken at mealtime. You have to check your written program instructions to find out exactly which, but it is possible that they may be taken either on an empty stomach or with food.

It's very common that you'd be taking the loosener supplements along with the bulldozer fiber cleanser on an empty stomach twice a day -- first thing in the morning, last thing at night; the digestive aids with each meal; and the mop-up killers with each meal.

It's very important that you drink a lot of water while you're doing this program. The items that you're taking tend to clean the bowel out and loosen debris and themselves absorb lots of water in order to do their job. Drinking eight glasses of water a day is almost a necessity for this to work. If you don't tolerate or digest fiber well, we might have to put you on NESS #12, #21, or #801 to help your body digest the fiber. You'll know if you're not digesting the fiber well if you become bloated, gassy, and/or constipated.

It's very common that people experience die-off reactions on Phase 2. This first part of Phase 2 is killing harmful organisms just as Phase I did. So, feeling ill is perfectly normal. You might not feel quite the same way as you did on Phase I. The type of die-off reactions that can occur on Phase 2 are similar to those in Phase I: flu-like symptoms. With that exception, it's more common that people will have gastro-intestinal upset, as opposed to some of the other Phase I symptoms. Rectal itching is very common, especially if you have worms or parasites. If you suddenly get rectal itching and have never had it before, that's a very good sign that your body is eliminating parasites and worms that were hidden deep in your system.

Generally speaking, while you're on this phase for a few days or maybe a week it's pretty common to feel flu-like; get gas; bloating; nausea; queasy; rectal itching; loss of appetite; and, perhaps, digestive upsets, This would not be unusual. It should pass after a period of time. If you feel ill on this phase or get constipated, you should call us. Constipation is the last thing we want on this phase. It's extremely important on this phase that your bowels be moving in order for you to get the results that are necessary. The reason for that is you're going to be killing unwanted organisms which are living in your system, and after they're killed we need your body to eliminate them so they're gone from your body. There's a certain amount of benefit to be had, or improvement to be had, from this phase by eliminating the organisms through cleansing. Cleansing has to mean that your bowels are moving. If your bowels are not moving, not much cleansing is going to occur, and we're not going to get the benefits that we need.

Following Phase 2, Part A, there is Phase 2, Part B. This is where we start to introduce friendly bacteria. There are three key products that we'll discuss on this phase. The first one is called FOS. FOS is a fruit sugar found in garlic, artichokes, bananas, and other fruits and vegetables that feeds friendly bacteria. It tends not to feed harmful bacteria; it seems to selectively feed only the friendly ones. Common friendly bacteria products that are used on this particular phase are Bifidofactor or Superdophilis. These are the name brands that are used because they are probably the most powerful and viable types of friendly bacteria known. They're referred to as the DDS strain, and we use them due to the fact that they're the best chance we have of getting a fast and thorough result. They are highly, highly potent products, and we with go with them as opposed to other ones to ensure a maximum, fastest result. We don't necessarily need to take a large dose of these. It's very common that a person will take a half of teaspoon of Bifidofactor in the morning, and perhaps a half teaspoon of Superdophilis at night while taking the FOS three times a day at a half-a-teaspoon dose. These should all be taken on an empty stomach because the acid in your stomach can kill these friendly bacteria. The FOS is the most important because the FOS will get into your intestinal tract and feed the friendly bacteria that you already have and get it to multiply. Even if you've been told from your test that you have no friendly bacteria, it's very unlikely the lab is implying that you have none whatsoever. You should have some, and whatever you do have will be fed by this FOS and will multiply.

It is very common when you begin Phase 2, Part B that you will get bloating, gas, and abdominal discomfort. That is due to taking the FOS, the Bifidofactor, and Superdophilis. The reason this seems to occur is that when the friendly bacteria starts to regrow, it produces gas and bloating. It does that because it's overrunning and wiping out the unfriendly bacteria. On Phase I and Phase 2, Part A, we're destroying the really harmful organisms living there. Surrounding those really harmful organisms --like Candida, parasites, worms, and things like that -- you have unfriendly bacteria or bacteria that really shouldn't be there, that is hanging out, taking up space, and occupying the area. The friendly bacteria that is multiplying from the FOS, Superacidophilis, and the Bifidofactor starts to overrun and crowd out this unfriendly stuff, and gas is produced. The simple thing to do when this happens, is to lower the dose of what you're taking. Cut the dose way back. You need to lower the dose down to whatever dose produces no reaction. Then slowly raise the dose until you can take the full dose that is written on your program. You may never get up to the full dose written on your program because you may not be able to tolerate the full dose, and it may actually not be necessary to get up to that full dose in order to get the results we want for you. The smartest and safest thing for you to do is simply raise the dose slowly to whatever you can tolerate and continue up on it until your next consultation, and then we'll see if it's worked at that dose anyway.

The last step of Phase 2 is where we repair the intestinal tract. This is done using certain vitamins and nutrients found in food that can first of all heal the intestinal tract of damage that is caused by the Candida. This is the "leaky gut" or the intentional permeability that we referred to before. This is also the phase where we can reduce inflammation that is in the intestinal tract.

The two main categories of supplements used on this part of the program are repair items and items that reduce inflammation. The purpose of repair is to stop arthritic symptoms or food reactions that are going on in the body. The key symptoms of intestinal permeability or "leaky gut" are allergic reactions to foods and also joint or arthritic symptoms. Some of these repair items can be taken with meals while others are taken on an empty stomach. You must consult your program to get the exact information. Repair items are highly individual, and I really could not give you much data about what you might be doing, because they are very individual. Suffice it to say that the main thing you should expect on this part of the phase is a reduction in food reactions or any arthritic or joint pain. Again – similar to what happened in Phase 2, parts A and B, you might experience gas or bloating or some change in your bowel movements. This is very common.

To summarize some of the key points or Phase 2:

1. Drinking water is extremely essential on this phase because your body is using the water to help clean your system out.

2. It's very common to feel or experience more Phase I-like reactions -- the die-off reactions, flu-like symptoms, etc. but it's more common that you'll get rectal itching or a change in the bowel movements or some type of digestive discomfort as the Candida is being killed, or the worms, parasites or whatever are being eliminated from your system.

3. It's very common when you take FOS, Superdophilis or Bifidofactor that are the friendly bacteria, that you'll experience gas, bloating and some discomfort as the friendly bacteria come back.

4. Whenever any of these products on any phase causes discomfort, you always lower the dose to whatever dose you can

tolerate, and then slowly raise it again.

5. Phase 2 generally is done in three sections, starting with Phase 2, Part A (nicknamed the mop-up section). This is where you are taking the mop-up Candida killers with the other bowel cleansers to help eliminate any remaining Candida, parasites, worms, or any harmful bacteria in the system.

6. The next section, Phase 2, Part B (the flora section), is where we introduce things to help bring back friendly bacteria into your system. And on that section you may experience bloating or gas, which is a signal that you need to lower the amounts of what you're taking to whatever dose you can tolerate without having those symptoms.

(PLEASE NOTE: The contents of this chapter are for informational purposes only. It is highly recommended that this program be conducted under the supervision of a qualified healthcare professional educated and certified in the Biamonte Method.)

Chapter 9

Phase 3: An interview

Interviewer: *So now that we've finished up Phase two, where do patients go from here?*

Dr. Biamonte: First, I like to congratulate my patients for completing Phases 0, 1, and 2! With time, effort, and the right guidance, major changes in health are possible, and as we enter into Phase 3, we are well on our way to achieving new levels of health, vitality, and wellbeing. Phase 3 of the program deals with energy and correcting any nutritional deficiencies which you may have incurred due to whatever infections that we were handling on Phase I.

On Phase 3, some specific tests are used. One is a blood test, and the other is a hair analysis. Depending on your specific situation, both of these tests may have been used, or perhaps only one of them. Both of these tests may have been sent to the Bio-Cybernetics Center for computer interpretation, or perhaps they were not, depending on your particular situation.

In a general sense, what is done is that the blood test is interpreted in a very special way. Back in the 1960s, Dr. Brockman began studying a wide variety of advanced medical textbooks to interpret blood tests in ways most physicians never thought possible. Dr. Brockman was also a learned expert in the blending of both Western and Eastern medicine and philosophies of healthcare. And now, fifty years later, his work has become an invaluable part the diagnostic arsenal used by the most elite of clinical nutritionists. Dr. Brockman's many years of exhaustive clinical observations have provided directions on how to effectively look at blood tests in a manner very different from those used by medical doctors. We use blood tests to get ideas of how well certain glands or organs or systems in your body are utilizing vitamins and minerals.

So now let's talk about hair analysis. It's been used since 1960, mainly by chiropractors and nutritionists, to determine mineral levels in your body. The hair -- being a dead tissue -- stores minerals. We want to know the storage in your body because storage is important for us to determine what level your body has to rely on. The amount of zinc stored in your hair reflects the amount of zinc stored in other glands, organs, and tissues in your body and gives us an idea of what the overall status in the body might be.

Blood levels of minerals are always being confused with hair levels of minerals by doctors and patients in trying to determine what is happening with you. If a doctor tells you that the iron in your blood is high, yet in the hair test it says that it's low, these mean two different things. Never expect the blood and the hair to agree on the same mineral. Many doctors and patients assume that if the blood says something is high and the hair says it's low, the hair is wrong, and everything is confused. Nothing could be further from the truth.

The hair and the blood can say totally opposite things -- or the same thing -- and these need to be interpreted by a skilled nutritionist who knows how to read the test to understand what it really means.

We expect the blood and the hair not to show the same values because they're showing different things. If a doctor tells you that the calcium levels in your blood are low, yet the nutritionist also says that the calcium in your hair is high, this means the same thing, even though it sounds like two different things. And the same thing is true of any other mineral we might talk about, if we're relating it to blood and hair together.

Let's look at this. If the levels of calcium in your blood are low, what this means is that your body is not using the calcium correctly or is not able to absorb it and send it where it needs to go in the body. If the levels of calcium in your hair are high, it means that the body is taking the calcium out of your blood and throwing it into tissues like your hair, or muscles, or arteries, and storing it there, and that's not where it's supposed to go. It's supposed to be evenly distributed through your blood, to muscles, glands, organs, and bones. So, high calcium levels in your hair will mean that your body is not utilizing calcium correctly and that you're actually deficient in calcium; so, of course, we expect to see it low in your blood. Blood shows transportation and hair shows storage. An analogy would be like this: if there were not many people riding on the bus, but many, many people waiting at the bus stop, this would show that the bus is basically empty and not moving many people around, but there are a lot of people there to be moved that are just standing there waiting at the bus stop.

In the blood, the calcium level is more like the bus. If there's not much calcium moving around in your blood, this is like not too many people on the bus being moved where they're supposed to go. If the calcium is high in your hair, it's the fact that there's too much calcium building up in certain spots of the body so that it's being stored there: it's locked up. And it's the same thing as having lots of people at the bus stop just hanging around waiting to be picked up. But of course these people are not getting where they're supposed to go and can't do their jobs -- just like the calcium in this situation can't do its job either. It's waiting around in the hair, or in tissues like the hair, just sitting there. It's very similar to having the old IRA accounts where you could put lots of money in, but not take it out. So, do you have lots of calcium? Yes, you do. Can your body USE the calcium and benefit from it? No, because you can't take it out, it's locked up in there.

This is the best analogy one can give. So, hair and blood are very important to the nutritionist to determine what's happening with you; however, they may not make sense to you or to your doctor unless you are skilled and have a degree or have studied exactly how to interpret these two tests.

The very first things that might be dealt with on your Phase 3 program are toxic metals. Toxic metals are extremely common in people. Many doctors don't think in terms of toxic metals these days because medical doctors are used to viewing things from the acute poison viewpoint -- meaning that someone has lead poisoning or arsenic poisoning and they have to be rushed to the hospital. While this does occur infrequently, *chronic toxicity* is more what people are experiencing and more what we're going to deal with on this phase.

One could easily say that four out of ten people living in any major city have a major overload of some kind of harmful, poisonous metal or mineral in their body. Yet they show no signs of acute poisoning, because that's simply not what they have. If someone goes out and eats lead paint or paint chips, or they go and take some harmful chemical in their body, they could get very sick and be tested and be found to have a very high level of some poisonous metal in their system. But that's not usually what happens. Usually a person accumulates mercury, copper, lead, or high levels of some other mineral very slowly in their body over a long period of time, and they never develop severe poisoning symptoms. Instead what they develop is many diseases or illnesses which have been in the medical literature, associated and proven to occur when your body builds up toxic metals. The science of toxic metals is fascinating; and, as a mystery, it's similar to the mystery of Candida.

The most common toxic metal can be copper, because most people have copper plumbing or copper pipes. It is very common that people will get excess build-up of copper in their system that can create all types of problems in your body. Copper is usually one of the first metals or minerals that we have to deal with eliminating from your system. Iron and lead and other minerals can also accumulate in your body. These are also very harmful.

The first thing we may want to do on your program if we find that you have toxic metals, is put you on special vitamins that help you eliminate these metals from your system. I can't emphasize this enough -- this is something you really have to understand -- when you have toxic metals in your body, and you start taking vitamins that remove the metals from your body, you are likely to feel ill. Just like on Phase I or Phase 3 if you have toxic metals. The most common symptoms that you might incur by removing toxic metals from your body are headaches, skin rashes, a metallic or metal taste in your mouth (which is a direct indication that metal is being eliminated from your system) or feeling sluggish or fatigued. These are very common symptoms of metal elimination from the body. Having aches and pains throughout the body is also very common when you remove toxic metals from the system.

These symptoms will go on until the metals have been fully eliminated from the body. That could take a few days, a few weeks, or a few months. Basically, as you're feeling sick your body is removing these toxic metals from your system. The more of these metals that are removed, the higher a dose on the vitamins you'll be able to tolerate, because there's not so much there to eliminate. So in the beginning, before you have eliminated these metals from your system, there's a lot to remove. Even a small dose of the vitamins may give you symptoms. But as you take the vitamins and you eliminate more and more of the metals, you can take a higher dose of the vitamins without getting sick because you don't have such an overload of the metal anymore in the body to push out. It's nothing to be worried or nervous about and very common for people eliminating heavy metals from their bodies. Just have patience and the symptoms will pass.

Many people who have arthritis or any type of joint or muscular or skeletal pain often have toxic metals. Women with severe PMS or difficulties conceiving or who have problems with their reproductive systems of any kind have toxic metals. There are many conditions in which a person may have toxic metals and where the only solution is to remove the metals. If you get scared and just give up because you can't tolerate taking the vitamins, you're never going to correct the condition. You can go to a chiropractor, nutritionist, medical doctor, witch doctors, psychics, voodoo from here to eternity, and you're never going to get rid of the condition until you remove those metals from your system. The only way to remove the metals is by taking targeted supplements, and taking them consistently until all the metals are gone.

What toxic metals will do to your body is prevent you from being able to absorb vitamins and minerals correctly. For example, you hear that zinc is good for the prostate, or zinc is good for PMS, and you want to handle your problem by taking zinc. That's fine. But if your body has high levels of cadmium, or nickel, or copper, these metals interfere with zinc in your body. You may take zinc, but not get any real benefit. In fact, you might feel bad taking the zinc, because zinc helps eliminate cadmium, nickel and copper from your system. The only way you're ever going to get the zinc to help your prostate or your PMS -- or whatever vitamin you're taking for whatever the condition -- is by getting that toxic metal out of your body so that the vitamin or mineral can work and do what it is that you want it to do.

This is something that I cannot stress enough. Many people who have gone on vitamin programs and have gotten bad reactions, have gotten these bad reactions because they had some type of poison in their system that the vitamin or mineral started to eliminate -- which is a good thing -- but the person, not knowing or understanding this, got scared and just dropped taking the vitamin or mineral and gave up. If you do that, you're never going to make it. And you're never going to get better. So please keep in mind that if you have any bad reactions from vitamins on this phase, it's because we're eliminating toxic metals from your system.

It's common that people who've had Candida, parasites, or Epstein-Barr virus to have an excess of copper and mercury in their body. This can come from the silver fillings in your mouth which are known and are scientifically proven to leak copper and mercury into your body, or it can just come from some source in your environment.

Mercury can occur in your body from eating too much fish; copper can come from your drinking water, or it can also come from certain medications. There are various ways you can get it; the main point is you need to know that someone who's had these chronic immune deficiencies usually is higher in copper or mercury or some harmful metal than someone who has not been suffering from these conditions like Candida, parasites, and Epstein-Barr.

The main problem most people have with their energy usually stems from the adrenal and the thyroid glands which are the main energy producers in the body. Many people may also have energy problems in their body due to reproductive organs that are deficient in nutrients. In a man, the reproductive organs would be the prostate and the testicles. In a woman, we're looking at the ovaries, the uterus. and the mammary glands (the glands in the breasts). Very commonly, women who've had chronic Candida have problems in their reproductive systems. Most medical doctors will tell you if you've had chronic yeast infections that it's very often linked to problems with your reproductive organs such as estrogen -- either too much estrogen or not enough. So usually every Phase 3 program for a woman who's had chronic yeast infections includes balancing out her reproductive system by taking the right vitamins. For a man, male hormones don't usually aggravate or cause a condition with yeast or parasites. But it's very common that in a man the reproductive organs might be attacked by the yeast or parasites. So attention may have to be given to those areas.

On Phase 3, the principal things that we're dealing with are glands and organs that involve energy. And in order to get these glands and organs to work better, we're going to use specific nutrients the tests indicate you're low in. Supplements are used on your program as they're shown needed by your test. The test may show that you need Vitamin A or Vitamin C or something, and this will be given to you on your program, and we will also give you a specific type of vitamin. We're not going to give you just any old type of Vitamin C or Vitamin A. From your tests and your medical history, we know exactly what type of that vitamin you might need. What I mean by "type" is that there are many kinds of Vitamin C and many kinds of Vitamin A or B-complex. While it may appear that there's only one kind of the vitamin, and it's all the same, that's not really true. These vitamins come in different forms and we can tell by your test which form your body will need or which form will be better in one person than another. So the type that we give you is very specific to you.

The minerals given in your program are, like the vitamins, given based on the deficiencies that show up on the tests. We may not give you some minerals you might be low in because if we do, it might cause something else to go out of balance. So, as you look through your tests, if you see that you're low in something, the reason you might not be getting it on your program at this time is because if you take it, it may actually cause some kind of upset in your body.

The protein concentrates that you're taking on this program are actual gland organ extracts. They're made by special companies that specifically raise animals for this exact purpose. The animals they use are bovine. These animals are specially raised for the purpose of later on taking their glands and organs, processing them in a special way -- like a freeze-dried method where the gland is taken raw from the animal -- the water and fat and all the poisons and toxins are removed from the gland of the animal, and it's sort of freeze dried and then made into a tablet. When your body takes this tablet, a good part of that protein is actually going to go to your own gland and help to rebuild or rejuvenate that gland by feeding it a similar protein to itself directly.

Many years ago, Native Americans told the white settlers that if they had a sick gland or organ, they should go and get an animal -- a deer, let's say -- and eat that same gland. So if the liver was sick, the Native peoples would tell the settlers to go get a deer and eat the liver. This probably sounded crazy and like voodoo to the medical people at that time. But in this century, we have found out why it works. The reason is that there is a compatibility between the proteins. It used to be taught in school that if you ate liver protein, your body wouldn't know any difference between that protein and steak and would treat it the same way. Eating that liver would not necessarily benefit your liver. Old, old medicine and wives' tales said otherwise. They said that if you had a problem, you should eat the same gland or organ that you were having a problem with, and that it would help you. Now different publications and medical journals and scientific journals have shown that when you do consume a protein form from a gland or organ, some of that protein does go to your own gland or organ and helps it. So, if you were to eat kidney, it would to some degree help your kidney. If you were to eat brain, to some degree it may help your brain tissue.

The pills we use on this program are specifically designed for this purpose and are more efficient than you going to a restaurant and ordering liver and onions to try to help your liver. About 20 to 30 percent of proteins that you're consuming in this pill form go directly to your gland and organ in order to rejuvenate it.

Many times you may also need to take an herb for the gland or organ because the herb has a stimulating effect. The protein pills have a rejuvenating or rebuilding feeding effect on the gland or organ, and the herbs tend to have a stimulating effect on the gland or organ.

If we find that you're not responding that well on the basic vitamin-mineral program, the next time that you come in, an herb or two may be added to specifically stimulate and wake up some of these glands and organs that are not functioning well.

Diet is very important on this phase because it uses a dietary strategy that addresses your exact metabolism. In the early 1970s, research done by nutritionists showed that everyone had a unique metabolism rate and that everyone's metabolism could be categorized in one of two categories: fast and slow metabolisms. People used these terms very often without really knowing what they were saying or using them correctly.

The definition of someone who has a slow metabolism is someone who's body does not burn up food into energy. Very specifically, it means somebody whose body cannot metabolize fats or proteins very well and cannot convert those things to energy quickly enough. Someone with a slow metabolism does very poorly when their body consumes fats. Fats tend to make the person feel sluggish, gain weight, and have very poor energy. If their metabolism is very slow and in very bad shape, their bodies will not be able to utilize protein very well. Usually such a person is constipated, tends toward cold hands and feet, dry skin, very bad energy levels, especially in the morning (very hard to get up). They may have low blood pressure. They usually tend to gain weight from the waist down, or in the thighs and hips as opposed to the upper body. The type of diet this person needs is a diet high in complex carbohydrates -- meaning grains, cereals, rice, pastas, noodles, beans, lentils, peas, and vegetables of all kinds, especially salads. Fruit is very important for this person's metabolism. And the person also needs to get lean protein in their diet. The best lean proteins are usually turkey, chicken, and fish. Red meats could be taken, but they should be trimmed of any fat and they should be very lean meats. Protein is extremely important for this person's type of metabolism because protein helps to raise your metabolism. If your metabolism is slow and you eat a meal that is high in protein and low in fat, it will stimulate your thyroid and adrenal and energy-producing glands to raise your metabolism and burn more calories over the next twelve hours. If you eat a meal that is high in fat, it will not do this. If you eat a meal that is high in carbohydrates or starch, it will not do this. Only protein does this.

The opposite of someone who has a slow metabolism is someone with a fast metabolism. A fast metabolism means a person's body is burning up foods into energy too quickly. When they eat, their body burns up the food very fast and then runs out of energy. Specifically, it is someone whose body burns up carbohydrates or starches very, very fast and then runs out of energy. These people, believe it or not, need to eat more oil or fats in their diets, because fats are slower-burning fuels. Only about 20 percent of the U.S. population has this kind of metabolism. I can tell you, as a side note, that since I've been a nutritionist, that this is a total amazement and mystery to many doctors and many nutritionists, that once in a while, you'll actually get a patient who does better on a high-fat diet, whose cholesterol drops and lowers on a high-fat diet, who loses weight easily on a high-fat diet.

There are actually several books written on this. Probably the best-known book on this subject is by Robert Atkins, who was a New York cardiologist and nutritionist. He had a radio show and wrote various books on the subject. In his books, Dr. Atkins talks about low carbohydrate diets with certain amounts of fat in the diet. Unfortunately, probably unknown to Dr. Atkins, he is specifically talking about a person who has this fast metabolism, which is only 20 percent of the population. That's about two out of every ten people you meet who have this metabolism.

People with fast metabolism have a particular body shape: their lower body is skinny, and their upper body is heavy. If you've ever seen pictures of the famous baseball player Babe Ruth or the famous actor-comedian W.C. Fields, you'll remember that these people had very skinny legs, practically no rear end (their buttocks was skinny) but from the waist up they were big and barrel-chested. And you may see or know people who have thin legs, thin thighs, not much of a backside -- from the waist down they're skinny, but from the waist up, the stomach, the chest, the shoulders, the neck, even the face -- they look fat. This is the shape of someone who has a fast metabolism. This is a person who will gain lots of weight very quickly, from starches, sugars, or alcohols; but, if they're put on a diet that is low in starches, sugars, or alcohols and that contains moderate amounts of proteins and healthy fats and are given vegetables that are not fattening, they'll lose weight easily and have very high energy.

Occasionally we'll find a person whose metabolism is fast; however, they may need to use the same diet as someone with a slow metabolism. This may be because the person's metabolism is exhausted. Sometimes due to stress, a person may lose certain minerals in their body which can speed their metabolism in a way that's giving them nervous energy and not giving them really pure energy. At the same time, due to the stress, their energy-producing glands like the adrenals and thyroid glands may become exhausted and go into a burn-out. We call this person an *exhausted fast metabolism type*. And we see more and more of these people as time goes by. This is due to the stress of high living and the demands that one encounters in life in these times. We find that people with this type of metabolism at one time may have had a legitimate fast metabolism, but now have exhausted and burned out, and they now need to treat themselves as though they were a slow metabolizer. They cannot use the diet that the fast metabolizer would normally use.

To summarize some of the key points on Phase 3:

1. The tests that are normally used to determine what is happening with your metabolism in order to raise your energy and your immune system are usually blood and hair tests From the results of these tests, you're going to be given a specific vitamin and mineral program, and that program will help you raise your energy and handle any nutritional deficiencies which you have due to having the active infection that was handled on Phase I.

2. It's very common that you may get bad reactions on Phase 3 in the beginning if you have toxic metals. Your nutritionist will most likely tell you if there is a toxic metal problem and will tell you to expect some kind of bad reaction as the metals are released from your system. Like the other earlier phases, the same holds true that you must lower the dose of whatever you're taking if you get a bad reaction, to the point where you're no longer getting that bad reaction. Stay at that dose for a few days or a week and then gradually raise the dose.

(PLEASE NOTE: The contents of this chapter are for informational purposes only. It is highly recommended that this program be conducted under the supervision of a qualified healthcare professional educated and certified in the Biamonte Method.)

Chapter 10

Phase 4:
An Interview

Interviewer: *So now we're at the final part of the program. Can you describe Phase 4?*

Dr. Biamonte: Phase 4 is solely dealing with your immune system and immune response on many different levels. The principal things we're concerned with on Phase 4 are to make sure the thymus gland, the spleen, and the lymphatic system are functioning properly. This is where a great deal of the immune response is generated. Another thing we're concerned with is liver function, as the liver does produce antibodies and does have an immune system response. We're also need to consider the adrenal glands, which have been strengthened or addressed on Phase 3.

On Phase 4 you could think that some of the Phase 2 technology has to be kept up or brought back if need be, in combination with the typical Phase 4 types of supplements. Speaking of which, the typical types of Phase 4 supplements primarily deal with those nutrients that help to generate an immune response and those herbs or nutrients which, when taken at the proper doses, stimulate the immune response.

If your Phase 4 program is broken up into two sections, Part A will deal with taking some nutrients for maybe a month or two which help to build and repair the immune system. Phase 4, Part B will deal with using specific herbs which stimulate the immune system.

On Phase 4, we can sometimes anticipate an energy increase. The reason for this is many times when the immune system is stimulated or functions at a higher level, there is more of an immune response and therefore higher energy. Sometimes on Phase 3, certain immune stimulants or immune-oriented supplements will be used to bring about higher energy. So this indeed could also happen on Phase 4, where we'll get an increased response of both the immune system and of energy.

On Phase 4, one should not necessarily expect bad reactions or expect any kind of side effects to occur. The only time that this is a consideration is if the person has known toxic metals in their system, and they have not all been fully eliminated on Phase 2 or Phase 3. In that case, you might have some kind of a toxic reaction. But the chances of this happening are slim. If there are toxic metals in the body, then a person may get a metallic taste in the mouth and other symptoms similar to that of Phase 3 when toxic metals are addressed.

Sometimes on Phase 4, a rash may break out, or pimples may break out. This is primarily due to the lymphatic system and the immune system cleansing itself. On Phase 3, when the reproductive organs are detoxifying themselves, it's common sometimes to get some type of a discharge from the reproductive organs or the skin such as a rash. This can also happen on Phase 4, as the organs of immune response start to detoxify themselves.

If this happens, a dry brush massage is very useful. This is a very simple technique that you can do yourself using what's known as a *dry brush*, which is available in health food stores. This helps to move the lymphatic system, push the poisons out of your skin, and increase the circulation. It's generally a good thing to do on Phase 4.

A sauna or steam bath is sometimes a good idea on Phase 4, as it allows the body to clean wastes and impurities out of the bloodstream and lymphatic system a bit more efficiently. If someone is getting rashes and pimples, sauna or steam bath is definitely a good idea.

Phase 4 is similar to Phase 3 in that it involves the interpretation of different kinds of tests, primarily a blood test and hair analysis. This is in order to determine what supplements are needed to start redeveloping the immune system. Sometimes a specific test for T-cells and B-cells (which is similar to the test given to HIV patients) may be done to determine the exact immune system requirements and provides results even more specific than we would normally achieve with the blood and hair tests. Sometimes test results are analyzed by the computer which does a whole analysis of the human body and gives us a read-out on all the different systems and how well they're working.

Sometimes on Phase 4 someone needs to do what we call a Vitamin C flush. A Vitamin C flush gives the system very, very high doses of Vitamin C to the point where it totally saturates the system, as part of bringing the immune system up. Essentially, when you're doing a Vitamin C flush, you're taking Vitamin C every hour, and you're recording the amount that you're taking. You're going to make a note of when you start developing a loose stool or diarrhea. If someone's taking 1000 mg of Vitamin C every hour for six hours, and in the sixth hour they have loose stools or diarrhea, that was 6000 mg of Vitamin C that was consumed. We then do a little simple arithmetic and arrive at the fact that was 6000 mg and then subtract 1000 mg, which would give you 5000 mg. What you would then do is every three hours take 5000 mg. It doesn't make any difference that it took six hours to have that occur; what we're concerned about is taking this same dose that produced the loose stool or diarrhea -- regardless of how many hours it took to accomplish that -- every three hours. Another example would be if someone took 1000 mg per hour for twelve hours, which would obviously be 12,000 mg. We would then subtract 1000 mg, we have 11,000 mg, and we're going to take that dose every three hours.

The person would continue to take this dose every three hours until a loose stool or diarrhea occurred again. If someone had done this for two days, let's say, taking this 11,000 mg dose every three hours, what they would do is now cut it down to 10,000 mg every three hours. And if they still had a loose stool or diarrhea they would cut it down to 9,000 mg. So every three hours they're cutting the dose down by 1000 to the point where they're not getting any loose stools or diarrhea. They would just continue this until their next appointment with the nutritionist or until they were told directly to discontinue this as far as their program. This is called the Vitamin C flush.

The reason that we achieve a loose stool when taking Vitamin C is that a loose stool signals that the body is totally saturated with Vitamin C and can no longer take anymore. This has been shown clinically to raise the immune response as high as possible from the Vitamin C.

Another program similar to this is sometimes done with the mineral germanium. For germanium to be effective, it's better to take it over the course of about four days or a week. The idea of this is that during that time you slowly raise the dose of the germanium. As an example, let's say a person started at 25 mg. They would then go to 50 mg, then 100 mg, then 150 mg, then 200 mg, then 250 mg. Let's say they stopped there; they would discontinue the germanium for two days, and then go back to 25 mg, then the next day 50 mg, then 100 mg, then 150 mg, then 200 mg, and then stop it again. It doesn't have to be done exactly like that, but that is the idea. The idea is to slowly raise the dose over a period of a few days, then discontinue it for two days and then go right back up again from a small dose. That is the most effective way to utilize it.

Vitamin A is another nutrient that sometimes has a little trick involved in taking it. With Vitamin A, sometimes we will use as much as 250,000 units of water-soluble A. This is a type of Vitamin A that generally doesn't accumulate in the liver for any long period of time. This 250,000 dose can be maintained for two or three weeks, after which case we drop the dose down to 50,000 units. It then can be brought up again to another 250,000 dose for another few weeks and then dropped again to 50,000 units for a week or so. So, one could conceivably do 250,000 units a day for two to three weeks and then take one to two weeks at 50,000 units. This again serves to stimulate certain parts of the immune system at a very high level.

Sometimes certain glandular concentrates from the thymus, lymphs, spleen, adrenals, and liver are also used in very high doses in order to generate and increase immune response. Sometimes they may be taken one tablet every hour. Many times, this will be used when the person has a severe cold or flu or when they feel extremely run down or are concerned or have evidence that they may be on the verge of a relapse, though on Phase 4. As a matter of fact, the Vitamin C flush, the germanium, Vitamin A and this hourly technique of taking these glandular concentrates may all be used if patients feel on the verge of a relapse. *On the verge of a relapse* means the patients feel like they're going to come down with something.

All of these techniques can be used by someone who is not on Phase 4 or who's not even on this program just to handle a cold or the flu. Generally speaking though, certain techniques are used on certain people or on certain types of illnesses, and we'll find that they work better. So, it's always better for the person to have a professional consultation with a nutritionist to determine this.

Echinacea, a commonly-used herb for the immune system, can also be used on Phase 4. When it is used, specifically when one feels a cold or flu coming on, the dose is 2 - 3 teaspoons, three times a day. After that initial high dose for that day, or maybe two or three days, the dose would be then dropped to maybe 1/2 teaspoon three times a day. Many times this is used on the onset of a cold or flu. Someone would take this massive dose and then cut it back for the duration of the program.

Phase 4 is a particular phase which unfortunately can be slow-moving, due to the fact that it takes so long to get yourself into such a mess where your immune system is so broken down. It may take a long time, but never nearly the amount of time it took to get you into this shape. It's generally thought that if a person had a condition like parasites, Candida, or a chronic viral condition, and they had this condition going on for 8 or 10 years, it may take 1/10 of that time to get them built up again. It wouldn't be unusual for Phase 4 to last a year or so before the person gets the full benefit from it. Phase 4 is the longest phase, generally speaking, because what we're now dealing with is the nitty-gritty of really rebuilding the immune response.

The major testing such as blood test or hair analysis done by independent laboratories outside the office are the tests that give us the data necessary to find out whether or not we're really getting the result that we need. And usually, because it's going to take some time for the program to really work and build up in the system, we then will only test the person in increments of three, four, or six months. Monthly testing at that point is no longer desirable or even workable.

Phase 4, when developed correctly by your nutritionist, is a maintenance program. A good and correct Phase 4 program may have some fiber supplements to keep the bowels moving and regular, some flora supplements to keep the bacteria correct, and digestive supplements to make sure you're digesting adequately. It may have some of the supplements from the Phase 2 repair section that have an immune-stimulating effect in the intestines, and it might also have certain supplements from the Phase 3 section which are energy boosters and could be immune boosters.

The primary work that will be done on Phase 4, though, is from the Phase 4 supplements. In some cases, it is possible that you may have very few supplements added to your Phase 4 program, and that your Phase 3 program brought in the majority of what was needed to accomplish the Phase 4 goal. This is possible and does happen to quite a few people, although it is not necessarily what we expect or anticipate. Usually when you get to Phase 4, you will be given a specific program of new supplements that rebuild the immune system.

It is possible with Phase 4 -- as it is with any other phase of the program -- that you can take all the tablets and any powders or liquids, put them all in a blender, and have the blender dissolve everything, and drink it! This is definitely desirable if you're like me and don't like taking a lot of pills. Actually, you may get better absorption and assimilation of your nutrients, and if you have loose stools or diarrhea, you may find that you don't have to take as many as on the program initially, because the tablets are breaking down and your system is getting what it needs from a smaller dose.

Generally speaking, whatever diet was given to you on Phase 3 to increase your metabolism or to decrease your metabolism if it was too fast, is generally the diet that will also be followed on Phase 4. The principal test that will determine your progress on Phase 4 will be the white blood count and the many individual white blood cells which are measured on a complete white blood count. Those are represented on a blood test as WBC (white blood count), a cenefils (a white blood cell that can indicate allergies), basofils (also a white blood cell that can indicate allergies), monocytes (which tell how well the liver is functioning), and the primary ones are neutrofils and leukocytes, which are very good indicators of infection in the body. On the other section of the blood test, the total globulin (which is a protein utilized by your immune system) also tells us how well the immune system is doing, as well as the albumin (which is another protein). A test called total bilirubin can give us some idea of how your thymus and liver are functioning, and they're definitely used to get an idea of the immune response in the system.

If any of these tests are out of the normal range, you're definitely going to want to follow up on them, and your nutritionist should instruct you to repeat the blood test in order to get an idea of how well those chemistries are doing.

In the hair analysis, some of the principal minerals which indicate the immune response in the body are zinc, copper, and iron. It's common in an immune-deficient person to have excessively low zinc and abnormally high copper. A very high or low iron also tells us something about how well the immune system is functioning. The mineral selenium, which shows in the hair, give us some idea of how well the body is responding to chemical toxins or odors and fumes and things in the environment that cause sensitivities. Toxic metals such as cadmium, mercury, lead, aluminum, and arsenic -- and we'd also include copper on this -- can also give us an idea of how well the immune response is doing. The lower these metals are, the better the immune response will be in the body.

(PLEASE NOTE: The contents of this chapter are for informational purposes only. It is highly recommended that this program be conducted under the supervision of a qualified healthcare professional educated and certified in the Biamonte Method.)

Chapter 11

Parasites: Types, Symptoms, Treatments, Associated Ailments, and Questions to Ask Yourself

Parasites are not a very happy subject. Most doctors believe that parasites only occur in Third World countries and cannot occur in the US. Parasites are truly "Merchants of Mayhem."

Why? Because:

1. They lie hidden in our bodies below our detection and awareness.
2. They are rarely revealed in even the best tests that seek to discover their presence in our bodies.
3. They create and cost a host of symptoms and medical conditions that are rarely attributed to them.

However, the issue of parasites has recently been getting some interesting press in several well know magazines.

In the words of National Geographic Magazine, our intestines and colons can become "a sinister world of monstrous creatures that feed on living flesh: parasites."

Discover Magazine published a feature article in its August 2000 issue that included the following statement:

> Every living thing has at least one parasite that lives inside or on it, and many, including humans, have far more. ...Scientists...are only just beginning to discover exactly how powerful these hidden inhabitants can be, but their research is pointing to a remarkable possibility: Parasites may rule the world. The notion that tiny creatures we've largely taken for granted are such a dominant force is immensely disturbing.

> ...We are collections of cells that work together, kept harmonized by chemical signals. If an organism can control those signals – an organism like a parasite – then it can control us. And therein lies the peculiar and precise horror of parasites.

The combination of environmental toxins, an unhealthy diet, and parasites poses a grave danger to humans. "In fact, parasites have killed more humans than all the wars in history", reported National Geographic in its award-winning documentary, *The Body Snatchers*.

Here are descriptions of the most common parasites found in ordinary people:

Hookworm (Ancylostoma duodenale)
The human hookworms include two nematode (roundworm) species, Ancylostoma duodenale, and Necator americanus. (Adult females: 10 to 13 mm (A. duodenale), 9 to 11 mm (N. americanus); adult males: 8 to 11 mm (A. duodenale), 7 to 9 mm (N. americanus). A smaller group of hookworms infecting animals can invade and parasitize humans (A. ceylanicum) or can penetrate the human skin (causing cutaneous larva migrans), but do not develop any further (A. braziliense, Uncinaria stenocephala). Eggs are passed in the stool and under favorable conditions (moisture, warmth, shade), larvae hatch in one to t wodays. The released rhabditiform larvae grow in the feces and/or the soil, and after five to 10 days (and two molts), they become filariform (third-stage) larvae that are infective. These infective larvae can survive three to four weeks in favorable environmental conditions. On contact with the human host, the larvae penetrate the skin and are carried through the veins to the heart and then to the lungs. They penetrate into the pulmonary alveoli, ascend the bronchial tree to the pharynx, and are swallowed. The larvae reach the small intestine where they reside and mature into adults. Adult worms live in the lumen of the small intestine

where they attach to the intestinal wall with resultant blood loss by the host. Most adult worms are eliminated in one to two years, but longevity records can reach several years.

Some A. duodenale larvae, following penetration of the host skin, can become dormant (in the intestine or muscle). In addition, infection by A. duodenale may probably also occur by the oral and transmammary route. N. americanus, however, requires a transpulmonary migration phase.

Geographic Distribution: The second most common human helminthic infection (after ascariasis). Worldwide distribution: mostly in areas with moist, warm climate. Both N. americanus and A. duodenale are found in Africa, Asia, and the Americas. Necator americanus predominates in the Americas and Australia, while only A. duodenale is found in the Middle East, North Africa, and southern Europe.

Roundworm (Ascaris lumbricoides)
Ascaris lumbricoides is the largest nematode (roundworm) parasitizing the human intestine. Immature or adult A.lumbricoides are sometimes passed in stools. Adult males measure 15 - 30 cm in length by 0.3 - 0.8 cm in diameter and have a ventrally curved tail; adult females measure 20 - 35 cm in length by 0.5 cm in diameter. Adult worms live in the lumen of the small intestine. A female may produce approximately 200,000 eggs per day which are passed with the feces . Unfertilized eggs may be ingested but are not infective. Fertile eggs embryonate and become infective after 18 days to several weeks depending on the environmental conditions (optimum: moist, warm, shaded soil). After infective eggs are swallowed, the larvae hatch, invade the intestinal mucosa, and are carried via the portal, then systemic circulation to the lungs . The larvae mature further in the lungs (10 to 14 days), penetrate the alveolar walls, ascend the bronchial tree to the throat, and are swallowed . Upon reaching the small intestine, they develop into adult worms. Between two and three months are required from ingestion of the infective eggs

to oviposition by the adult female. Adult worms can live one to two years.

Geographic Distribution: The most common human helminthic infection. Worldwide distribution. Highest prevalence in tropical and subtropical regions, and areas with inadequate sanitation. Occurs in rural areas of the southeastern United States.

Pinworm (Enterobius vermicularis)
The nematode Enterobius vermicularis (previously Oxyuris vermicularis) also called human pinworm. (Adult females: 8 -13 mm, adult male: 2 - 5 mm.) Humans are considered to be the only hosts of E. vermicularis. A second species, Enterobius gregorii, has been described and reported from Europe, Africa, and Asia. For all practical purposes, the morphology, life cycle, clinical presentation, and treatment of E. gregorii is identical to E. vermicularis.

Eggs are deposited on perianal folds. Self-infection occurs by transferring infective eggs to the mouth with hands that have scratched the perianal area. Person-to-person transmission can also occur through handling of contaminated clothes or bed linens. Enterobiasis may also be acquired through surfaces in the environment that are contaminated with pinworm eggs (e.g., curtains, carpeting). Some small number of eggs may become airborne and inhaled. These would be swallowed and follow the same development as ingested eggs. Following ingestion of infective eggs, the larvae hatch in the small intestine and the adults establish themselves in the colon . The time interval from ingestion of infective eggs to oviposition by the adult females is about one month. The life span of the adults is about two months. Gravid females migrate nocturnally outside the anus and oviposit while crawling on the skin of the perianal area . The larvae contained inside the eggs develop (the eggs become infective) in four to six hours under optimal conditions. Retroinfection, or the migration of newly hatched larvae from the anal skin back into the rectum, may occur but the frequency with which this happens is unknown.

Geographic Distribution: Worldwide, with infections more frequent in school- or preschool- children and in crowded conditions. Enterobiasis appears to be more common in temperate than tropica l countries. The most common helminthic infection in the United States (an estimated 40 million persons infected).

Schistosoma

Schistosomiasis is caused by digenetic blood trematodes. The three main species infecting humans are Schistosoma haematobium, S. japonicum, and S. mansoni. Two other species, more localized geographically, are S. mekongi and S. intercalatum. In addition, other species of schistosomes, which parasitize birds and mammals, can cause cercarial dermatitis in humans.

Eggs are eliminated with feces or urine. Under optimal conditions, the eggs hatch and release miracidia, which swim and penetrate specific snail intermediate hosts. The stages in the snail include two generations of sporocysts and the production of cercariae . pon release from the snail, the infective cercariae swim, penetrate the skin of the human host , and shed their forked tail, becoming schistosomulae. The schistosomulae migrate through several tissues and stages to their residence in the veins. Adult worms in humans reside in the mesenteric venules in various locations, which at times seem to be specific for each species. For instance, S. japonicum is more frequently found in the superior mesenteric veins draining the small intestine, and S. mansoni occurs more often in the superior mesenteric veins draining the large intestine. However, both species can occupy either location and they are capable of moving between sites, so it is not possible to state unequivocally that one species only occurs in one location. S. haematobium most often occurs in the venous plexus of bladder , but it can also be found in the rectal venules. The females (size 7 - 20 mm; males slightly smaller) deposit eggs in the small venules of the portal and perivesical systems. The eggs are moved progressively toward the lumen of the intestine (S. mansoni and S. japonicum) and of the bladder and ureters (S. haematobium), and are eliminated with feces or urine, respectively. Pathology of S. mansoni and S. japonicum schistosomiasis includes Katayama fever, hepatic perisinusoidal egg granulomas, Symmers' pipe stem periportal fibrosis, portal hypertension, and occasional embolic egg granulomas in brain or spinal cord. Pathology of S. haematobium schistosomiasis includes hematuria, scarring, calcification, squamous cell carcinoma, and occasional embolic egg granulomas in brain or spinal cord.

Human contact with water is thus necessary for infection by schistosomes. Various animals, such as dogs, cats, rodents, pigs, hourse and goats, serve as reservoirs for S. japonicum, and dogs for S. mekongi.

Geographic Distribution: Schistosoma mansoni is found in parts of South America and the Caribbean, Africa, and the Middle East; haematobium in Africa and the Middle East; and S. japonicum in the Far East. Schistosoma mekongi and S. intercalatum are found focally in Southeast Asia and central West Africa, respectively.

Tapeworm

The cestodes (tapeworms), Taenia saginata (beef tapeworm), and Taenia solium (pork tapeworm). T.saginata may measure 9 m (27 ft), whereas T.solium may reach 6 m (18 ft). Taeniasis occurs when raw or undercooked unfrozen beef (T.saginata) or pork (T.solium) are eaten. T. solium can also cause cysticercosis.

Humans are the only definitive hosts for Taenia saginata and Taenia solium. Eggs or gravid proglottids are passed with feces; the eggs can survive for days to months in the environment. Cattle (T. saginata) and pigs (T. solium) become infected by ingesting vegetation contaminated with eggs or gravid proglottids. In the animal's intestine, the oncospheres hatch, invade the intestinal wall, and migrate to the striated muscles, where they develop into cysticerci. A cysticercus can survive for several years in the animal. Humans become infected by ingesting raw or undercooked infected meat . In the human intestine, the cysticercus develops over two months into an adult tapeworm which can survive for years. The adult tapeworms attach to the small intestine by their scolex and reside in the small intestine . Length of adult worms is usually 5 m or less for T. saginata (however it may reach up to 25 m) and 2 - 7 m for T. solium. The adults produce proglottids which mature, become gravid, detach from the tapeworm, and migrate to the anus or are passed in the stool (approximately six per day). T. saginata adults usually have 1,000 to 2,000 proglottids, while T. solium adults have an average of 1,000 proglottids. The eggs contained in the gravid proglottids are released after the proglottids are passed with the feces. T. saginata may produce up to 100,000 and T. solium may produce 50,000 eggs per proglottid respectively.

Geographic Distribution: Both species are worldwide in distribution. Taenia solium is more prevalent in poorer communities where humans live in close contact with pigs and eat undercooked pork. Both species are very rare in Muslim countries.

Whipworm (Trichuris trichiura)
The nematode Trichuris trichiura, also called the human whipworm. The adult female measures about 35 - 50 mm in length, and the male about 30 - 45 mm. The unembryonated eggs are passed with the stool. In the soil, the eggs develop into a 2-cell stage, an advanced cleavage stage, and then they embryonate; eggs become infective in 15 to 30 days. After ingestion (soil-contaminated hands or food), the eggs hatch in the small intestine, and release larvae that mature and establish themselves as

adults in the colon. The adult worms (approximately 4 cm in length) live in the cecum and ascending colon. The adult worms are fixed in that location, with the anterior portions threaded into the mucosa. The females begin to oviposit 60 to 70 days after infection. Female worms in the cecum shed between 3,000 and 20,000 eggs per day. The life span of the adults is about one year.

Geographic Distribution: The third most common roundworm of humans. Worldwide, with infections more frequent in areas with tropical weather and poor sanitation practices, and among children. It is estimated that 800 million people are infected worldwide. Trichuriasis occurs in the southern United States.

General Symptoms of a Parasitic Infection

Acute parasite infection is usually characterized by greater or lesser abdominal distress and diarrhea, often urgent and attended by burning sensations and tremendous fluid loss. Only rarely is there any visible evidence of infection. Moreover, many laboratories fail to detect the presence of parasites even when presented with specimens from infected persons. It is therefore sometimes necessary for the patient to determine whether infection is likely and to self-administer some remedy since allopathic medicine requires a diagnosis before prescriptions can be written.

Once a condition has moved from acute to chronic, there may be alternating periods of constipation and diarrhea, abdominal distention and bloating, intestinal cramping followed by burning sensations, and the sudden urge to eliminate. Generally, there is malabsorption of nutrients, especially fatty foods. Irritable bowel syndrome, blood sugar fluctuations, sudden food cravings, and extreme emaciation or overweight are all possible symptoms; but, as stated, not necessarily proof of parasitic infection. Itching is a possible clue to infection, especially among children; however, the absence of itching does not mean there is no infection. The itching tends to be worst where there is moisture: nose, eyes, ears, and of course the anus. Skin sensitivity is also common: rashes, eczema-like conditions, and even serious eruptions.

Many parasites affect the nervous system and give rise to sleep disorders, such as insomnia. In children, hyperactivity is common, but adults may have symptoms ranging from depression to anxiety. Some parasites affect the brain and memory.

In our practice we have had many children whose seizures improved greatly after doing a parasite elimination program. In fact, the mother of one patient referred over 10 other patients that she had met in her child's neurologist's waiting room. In time all were able to obtain similar improvements and their neurologist was able to discontinue their medications.

In short, the part of the body affected depends on where the parasites have invaded: blood, intestines, liver, pancreas, kidneys, brain, etc. To make infection even more difficult to determine, add to this scenario the fact that many, if not most, parasites migrate so the symptoms could change depending on where the parasites are at any given time.

The 2 Most Common Ailments Associated with Parasites

Diseases caused by parasites are fairly common in children who play in dirt where worms and other parasites live. The parasites often go from the ground into a child's body when the child puts his dirty hands into his mouth. Parasites also get into children's bodies when they kiss or hug or play with pets who are infected worms or have ticks on their bodies. And finally, parasites may enter the body when an infected insect, like a mosquito carrying the malaria parasite, bites someone's skin.

Here's how the infection caused by one of four kinds of malarial parasite functions. It comes about when a person is bitten by a mosquito that is infected with the parasite. During the first week of malaria, the patient will have attacks of fever, headaches, and chilly sensations. Then, during the weeks afterward, the patient may feel fine one day, and the next day have a high fever and severe chills lasting for a few hours. Then, the patient will break out in a great sweat. This situation continues with one day high fever and chills, the next day no fever or chills. The mosquitoes that carry the malaria parasites breed primarily in the humid, hot climate of the tropics and subtropics. They are seldom found in temperate regions.

The diagnosis of malaria is made by taking a little sample of the patient's blood and examining it under a microscope. On examination, the malaria parasite will be found. Malaria attacks may go on for many weeks or months if treatment isn't given. Fortunately, there are several excellent medications to control malaria, but they must be given over a long period of time in order to cure the condition. To prevent this disease, people in areas where malaria exists should take anti-malarial pills every day, and they should protect themselves against being bitten by mosquitoes.

Amebic dysentery

An ameba is a single-celled animal organism that may cause diseases in children. The most common of such diseases is dysentery caused by Endameba histolytica. Amebic dysentery is a form of diarrhea caused by a tiny one-celled animal parasite called the ameba. A child with amebic dysentery will have crampy pains in his abdomen; many watery; loose bowel movements; loss of appetite; loss of weight, and anemia. The diagnosis of this condition is made by examining the stool in a laboratory and seeing the ameba parasite under a microscope. Luckily, there are excellent medicines to kill the parasite and cure the child. To prevent amebic dysentery, children must be very clean about their bodies and their eating habits. Also, if children aren't careful, they may spread the infection to other members of their families.

Ailments Reported By Other Health Practitioners

Dr. Hulda Clark: "I have seen that eczema is due to roundworms. Seizures are caused by a single roundworm, Ascarts, getting into the brain. Schizophrenia and depression are caused by parasites in the brain. Asthma is caused by Ascaris in the lungs. Diabetes is caused by the pancreatic fluke of cattle, Eurytrema. Migraines are caused by the threadworm, Strongyloides. Acne rosacea is caused by a Leishmania. Much human heart disease is caused by dog heartworm, Dirofilaria. And the list goes on and on." Two main kinds of arthritis are recognized clinically, osteoarthritis and rheumatoid arthritis. In osteoarthritis, the joints have bacteria living in the deposits left there. In rheumatoid arthritis the bacteria come from larger parasites -- wormlets actually living in these joints. The worms are the common little roundworms whose eggs hatch into microscopic wormlets that travel.

Suzanne M. Skinner, PhD., RNC, HHP, CH is a nutritionist and holistic health practitioner: "In my practice, I always find parasites and worms associated with the following diseases: Diabetes, hypoglycemia, juvenile diabetes, anorexia, asthma, depression, anemia, chronic fatigue syndrome, AIDS, cancer, tumors, anorexia, bulimia, colitis, epilepsy, hyper-activity syndromes, learning disabilities, baldness, prostate trouble, appendicitis (the appendix is a favorite place for parasites), elevated white blood counts, Hodgkin's disease, Multiple Sclerosis, psoriasis, some eczemas, leukemia, lymphoma, arthritis, leprosy, ulcerative colitis, low hemoglobin, poor blood quality, iron deficiencies and most bowel disorders."

Contagious Canine Cancer Spread by Parasites

According to Charles Q. Choi, Special to Live Science, dogs have a form of sexually transmitted cancer that for 2,000 to 2,500 years has apparently spread via contagious tumor cells that escaped from their original body and now travel around the world as parasites. These cells are the oldest cancers known to science thus far and could shed light on how cancers survive and evade the immune system.

Lung Disease in The Tropics by Om P Sharma (Page 33) explains that Parasites migrate through the lungs as part of their life cycle.

The Arthritis Center of Riverside has been established since 1988. Al Robert Franco, MD, FACR, the founder and Medical Director, has indicated that the interrelationship between infections and rheumatic diseases has been discussed in the medical literature for decades. Microorganisms that cause bone and joint disease include bacteria, Mycoplasmas, viruses, fungi, and parasites. Parasites have been associated with joint and bone lesions. These include protozoa, flat worms, and round worms.

In their "Dysbiosis," Eugene Zampieron, ND and Ellen Kamhi PhD RN, write that the proliferation of "unfriendly" microorganisms, including bacteria, yeast, fungi and parasites, is not widely recognized by conventional medicine as a cause of arthritis. Yet, these organisms are present in a large majority of people who suffer from muscle and joint pains. "Molecular Mimicry" is an additional complication, which arises when organisms in the gut camouflage themselves to resemble human tissue to escape detection by the immune system. When the immune system eventually makes antibodies to the bacteria, it also begins to make antibodies to the similarly structured human tissue, leading to an autoimmune cascade.

Dr. Ronen Arai, Senior Fellow in Gastroenterology at the University Of Miami School Of Medicine in Miami, Florida, writes that There are many kinds of parasites that can invade the liver, causing acute and/or chronic liver damage depending on the type of parasite involved. Some clues to the type of parasite affecting your friend's mother may lie in her eating habits, as well as her ethnicity. One parasitic disease, trichinosis, arises from eating undercooked meat. In this disease, parasites can affect the bile ducts draining the liver, leading to right-sided abdominal pain, fever, jaundice, and an enlarged liver. While the patient may be acutely ill, anti-parasitic drug therapy will usually lead to resolution. Trichinosis does not typically lead to cirrhosis.

Another parasitic infestation, clonorchiasis, is linked to eating raw fish. This infection is most common in Asia. It is a more chronic disease than trichinosis, and patients usually do not experience symptoms until long after the initial parasitic infection. Symptoms include right-sided abdominal pain and jaundice. Imaging studies of the abdomen and liver may reveal evidence of the obstruction of the bile ducts draining the liver, a situation that may be mistaken for cancer of the bile ducts. Ironically, by causing chronic inflammation in the bile ducts, long-standing clonorchiasis sometimes actually leads to bile-duct cancer. Although the disease is usually diagnosed when bile-duct obstruction occurs, if it is not detected soon enough, scarring of the liver (cirrhosis) may have already occurred.

Finally, cirrhosis of the liver can be a direct result of parasitic disease. In a condition called schistosomiasis, parasites travel to the liver and settle in the liver's small veins. After some time, scarring (cirrhosis) occurs as a result of the inflammation and the body's attempt to fight the infestation. This parasite is acquired via skin exposure, usually from wading barefoot in fresh water in Asian countries.

Questions to Ask Yourself!

DO YOU GRIND YOUR TEETH AT NIGHT?

Teeth grinding is often caused by a calcium deficiency. However, parasites have been found to block the absorption of calcium which can then lead to the calcium deficiency.

DOES YOUR CHILD SUFFER FROM SEIZURES?

In our practice, we have been alarmed by the number of young children suffering with seizures who have come to us and by the number of these children who have improved after doing a parasite cleanse! The improvements range from 50 percent to 100 percent.

DO YOU HAVE SEIZURES OR EPILEPSY?

According to Dr. Thomas Brooks, author of "The Essentials of Medical Parasitology," neurological disorders occur when the central nervous system is invaded by parasites. The tiny larva from the pork tapeworm can get into the brain. If they get into the right spots, seizures and epilepsy will occur.

DO YOU HAVE RECTAL ITCH THAT WORSENS AT NIGHT?

This is caused by pinworms or "seat worms." The crawling of the worm on the perianal area produces the intense itching. When you scratch yourself the parasites eggs get on your fingers! Parasites become more active at night when they deposit their eggs, particularly during a full moon. During these times their metabolisms speed up and they release more toxic wastes. These eggs deposit their eggs on pajamas and linens.

DO YOU HAVE SHORTNESS OF BREATH?

The eggs from roundworms travel through your entire system and go through different stages before settling in the intestines. At one of their stages, they settle in the lungs. If too many larvae settle in the lungs, shortness of breath and lung inflammation can result.

DO YOU HAVE LIVER, JAUNDICE, OR BILE DUCT PROBLEMS?

Roundworms have been known to leave the intestines and go into the liver or bile duct causing obstructions. They can also cause more serious liver problems and disease.

DO YOU HAVE CHRONIC VAGINAL YEAST OR ITCHING THAT DOESN'T

RESPOND TO TREATMENT?

Parasites can live in the vaginal area. Even the kind that you can see with the naked eye! Parasites can cause yeast and keep it there! They can cause itching and inflammation by directly attacking the mucus lining of the vaginal area. If you ever have strings of mucus from the vaginal area or in your stool, look closely as it may be a worm. Look for something that looks like a head or for intestines running the length of its body.

DO YOU FEEL AS IF SOMETHING IS BITING OR CRAWLING UNDER YOUR SKIN?

As gross as it may sound, there are parasites that can crawl under different layers of skin and in the lymphatic system. They can also literally bite at skin and mucus membranes. Some people feel this at night while lying in bed and particularly in the rectal area.

DO YOU GET UNCONTROLLABLE FOOD CRAVINGS?

Many parasites love and crave sugar. They can rob you of so much of your nourishment that your blood sugar can crash causing hypoglycemia. Some parasites love fat and grease and can cause you to crave chips, fries, and fast foods!

DO YOU HAVE UNEXPLAINED BONE LOSS?

Certain parasites eat the calcium right off your bones! These parasites are microscopic and hard to locate. If you are having unexplained bone loss at an early age, this could be why.

DO YOU GET UNEXPLAINED FEVERS AND DIARRHEA?

Many of us think of fever and diarrhea as being caused by viruses. However, if your symptoms began particularly after swimming in a river, lake, or stream, you may have contracted a parasite called Guardia. Giardia commonly causes fever and diarrhea. It occurs from time to time in New York public water supplies.

DO YOU HAVE CHRONIC DERMATITIS COVERING LARGE AREAS OR MOST OF YOUR BODY?

Reports from my own office and from colleagues of mine show that people with severe chronic dermatitis are infected with many parasites. Dramatic and miraculous improvements have occurred by doing parasite cleansing.

HAVE YOU BEEN DIAGNOSED WITH ANEMIA OR HAVE YOU BEEN CHRONICALLY TIRED FOR YEARS AND NOTHING HAS HELPED?

Some parasites called hookworms can attach themselves to the lining of the intestines and bite into our blood vessels drinking our blood. Chronic hookworm disease can cause extreme and chronic anemia. Cats are a common source of these worms. These worm eggs can easily get into your system after you contact your pet!

HAVE YOU HAD A RASH OR ITCHY SKIN AND THEN A MONTH LATER HAD FEVER, CHILLS, COUGH AND MUSCLE ACHES THAT WON'T GO AWAY?

If so, you may have Schistosomaisis. This is an illness caused by your body's reaction to the eggs of worms. You can get it by swimming in water that has had certain types of snails living in it. These parasites absorb through the skin. The parasite is normally found in Africa, the Middle East, the Caribbean, Latin America, and Southeast Asia.

DO YOU HAVE HAIR LOSS, ROUGH SKIN OR A TENDENCY TO FLUSH AROUND THE FACIAL REGION?

If so, you may have a parasitic mite known as demodex brevis or demodex folliculorum. This parasite can live in the hair follicle. It sucks out the nutrients at the root of the hair. The follicle becomes enlarged and infected causing loss of hair and inflammation. When living on the skin, it feeds on nutrients in the sebaceous glands, they become infected and inflamed and the skin may then thicken. Acne Rosacea can also be caused by this parasite.

DO YOU GET DIARRHEA, GAS, STOMACH CRAMPS, AND NAUSEA, VOMITING, FATIGUE, WEIGHT LOSS AND LOW GRADE FEVER FOR

SEVERAL WEEKS THEN GOES AWAY AND THEN RETURNS?

If yes, you may have a parasite that has been found on raspberries called cyclosporiasis. It came into this country from Guatemala on raspberries. There were two large out breaks of it in May and June of 1996. It is very hard to diagnosis. If you feel you have this, please notify the Centers for Disease Control in Atlanta, Georgia.

DO YOU HAVE CHRONIC ABDOMINAL PAIN, WEAKNESS, LOSS OF WEIGHT, NAUSEA, AND DIZZINESS?

If yes, you may have a tapeworm that comes from eating rare beef. This tape worm takes up to three months to grow into an adult after it's ingested. This worm can grow from 13 to 39 feet in length. It is considered the second largest tape worm.

HAVE YOU HAD CONSTIPATION AND CHRONIC ANEMIA?

There is a fish tape worm that can reach 33 feet in length! In fact, it can get so big that it can cause colon blockage which will appear to you as constipation. It can cause anemia, interfering with B12 absorption. Researchers Davies and Goldsmidt in 1978 also found that roundworms can cause intestinal obstructions. This happens when many roundworms "ball up" into one big mass.

DO YOU SUFFER FROM UNEXPLAINED CONVULSIONS OR FITS?

According to Geoffrey Lapage the author of "Animals Parasitic in Man," poisonous substances produced by this same beef tapeworm can cause unexplained convulsions. The worm can even damage the intestines causing ulceration's and infections.

Pharmaceuticals and Parasites

W. Peters wrote in the Institute of Medicine, Division of International Health, Pharmaceuticals for developing countries. (Conference proceedings, Washington, D.C., January 29-31, 1979) Washington, D.C., National Academy of Sciences, 1979. (IOM-79-001) p. 59-82, "Simple improvements in personal hygiene, in water supplies, in disposal of excreta, and in housing do more to reduce or even eliminate many parasitic diseases than the use of specific anti-parasitic drugs. Also needed in the future will be new and better drugs to help prevent and control many parasitic conditions. Full collaboration of the pharmaceutical industry is essential if new anti-parasitic drugs are to be discovered. It is also necessary to strengthen the facilities for clinical trials of new drugs as they emerge."

In a Medical Letter on the CDC & FDA (2000-11-12) called "Economic Realities Depleting Arsenal" November 12th, 2000, "While resistance may be reducing the effectiveness of our medicine chest, we have another force to fear: economics. Many drugs still effective against parasitic diseases are either no longer available, no longer manufactured, or in danger of being pulled from the market simply because they are not economically viable, say researchers from the Baylor College of Medicine and the U.S. Centers for Disease Control and Prevention (CDC) at a presentation during the annual meeting of the American Society of Tropical Medicine and Hygiene in October 2000. Parasites are a very common cause of disease in the world but because there is no market for anti-parasitic."

The Secret of an Effective Parasite Program

Herbal treatments for parasitic infections are widely available and have been historically effective if used correctly. Over a 20 year period, I have personally used and tested dozens of formulas and products. Freshness and quality of the herbs are often more important than the formulation. One can have an amazing formula, but if the quality of the herbs are poor, and if they are so old as to render the active ingredients, than the product will not provide satisfactory results.

When a package containing herbs is first opened, there should be a strong aromatic smell to the product. The product should not look oxidized, moldy, or be disintegrating. Herbs should not smell musty, moldy, or like a chemical. Herbs should smell fresh, vibrant, and grassy or flowery depending on the herb.

Adult parasites, commonly seen with the naked eye are typically referred to as *worms*. Worms may also be called helminthes, particularly in medical terminology when referring to parasitic worms, especially the Nematode (roundworms) and Cestoda (tapeworms). Hence "helminthology" is the study of parasitic worms. When an animal, such as a dog, is said to "have worms," it means that it is infested with parasitic worms, typically roundworms or tapeworms. Worms in general are easy to kill using herbs. The true challenge is destroying the eggs that are being constantly laid. The eggs are almost impossible to kill due to the frequency with which they are produced. As the herbs kill the adults, the eggs they have laid begin to hatch. Mother Nature loves all her babies, not just us. So the protocol must be carried out long enough to kill the eggs that hatch and to permeate the eggs as they are laid in order to kill them. The length of time is typically agreed upon as being 30 - 90 days. If one does not complete the cleanse in that time period, the products being used are either inferior or the patient is being reinfected. Also antioxidant vitamins must be avoided during the 30, 60 or 90 cleanse period. Vitamins will serve as antidotes for the herbal medicines and protect the parasites from their effects. Why bother doing a parasite cleanse if you are going to revive them with vitamins

Traditional Herbal and Botanical Treatments for Parasites

There are many herbal-botanicals that have been used for microscopic parasite infections (protozoa) and for intestinal worm infections (helminthes). In this section, we are going to concentrate on the key herbs that are generally agreed upon by most herbalists as being the most important for the elimination of helminthes. Keep in mind that there are other adjunctive substances used besides the ones mentioned here!

Black Walnut Hulls

Organically grown green black walnut extract is what is preferred by most practitioners. It is considered a powerful vermifuge agent for treating parasite conditions. Green black walnut extract is made from organically grown, green black walnut hulls. It is produced in a special way that maximizes its potency. Green black walnut extract greatly assists the removal of parasites from extra cellular fluids, such as the blood and lymph, and in organs such as the liver, kidneys, brain, heart, and intestinal tract. Several species of walnut tree grow in the United States. Two of these are native to the East: the black walnut and the butternut, also called the white walnut. Black walnut trees grow in forests from Massachusetts to Florida and west to Texas. They are hardy trees that are grown mainly for their lumber. The nuts also are harvested and sold. They have a distinctive and rich flavor, but their shell is hard and thick. Black walnut wood is dark purplish-brown with a fine grain and luster. It is valuable for interior finishing, furniture, and gunstocks. This wood is becoming rare. The Black Walnut Hull contains a number of active ingredients, of which the most important are juglone, tannins, and iodine. Juglone is a brown constituent of the black walnut hull, leafs, bark, and even roots. It is called a *phytotoxic allelochemical*. *Phytotoxic* means that it kills plants, and *allelochemical* means that the black walnut tree produces this chemical to keep other plants from growing around it. You may have noticed that vegetation under black walnut trees is rather scarce, and this is the reason. Since yeast and fungus in humans are also plants, it has been conjectured that it will work against fungus as well, and it has been described as an anti-fungal in many herbal reference books. There is some scientific evidence also. Whether juglone works against parasitic infections is matter of scientific discussion. However, the NIH (National Institute of Health) writes: "Crushed unripe walnut hulls have been used for generations in various types of folk medicine [...] to treat fungal, bacterial or viral infections such as herpes or warts. External applications of walnut also kill ringworm, and Chinese herbalists use this substance to kill tapeworm." Since we suspect that juglone is the most important ingredient in black walnut hull tincture, and since it can quickly oxidize rendering the tincture less potent, we have developed a laboratory method to monitor the concentration of juglone in our black walnut hull tincture.

Tannins act as a defense mechanism in plants against pathogens, herbivores, and hostile environmental conditions. The antihelminthic properties of tannins have been shown in scientific studies. Tannins are described to be antibacterial, anticancer, antidiarrheic,an tihepatotoxic, chelator, antihypertensive, anti-tumor, cancer preventive, and anti-ulcer. Unfortunately, little scientific information can be found about tannins. Iodine is widely used as an antiseptic in medicine. It works by attaching itself to the pathogenic bacteria and thereby killing them.

Artemisia Annua

The species of wormwood known as Artemisia annua has been used in traditional Chinese medicine for the treatment of fevers and malaria for many centuries. The active antimalarial compound known as artemisinin was isolated by Chinese researchers in the early 1970s. Since then, research has focused on artemisinin and its semi-synthetic derivatives such as artemether and artesunate. These drugs have become established as safe and effective antimalarial drugs that have particular value in the treatment of chloroquine-resistant parasites. However, a group of German scientists have focused their research effort on the use of the whole herb, particularly when taken as an infusion with boiling water. The motivation behind this research is to understand the value of the traditional use of Artemisia annua for the treatment of malaria, because this application could be readily adopted in poor countries such as many Africa nations where the semi-synthetic drugs are relatively expensive.

Artemisia annua interacts with the iron found in cancer cells, the parasite, or the yeast organism. This creates "oxidative stress" or "free radical" activity in the parasite, cancer cell or Candida/ yeast cell, and the oxidative stree which kills them! Artemisia annua is most effective against roundworms, hookworms, whipworms, and pinworms. Artemisia contains the toxins thujone and isothujone which are the components that kill parasites. It also contains santonin which is known as a remedy for parasitic diseases. The second most bitter herb known to man, Artemisia annua also contains sesquiterpene lactones which work similarly to peroxide by weakening the parasites membranes thereby killing them. A research team investigated the clinical efficacy of an Artemisia annua tea in the treatment of subacute malaria in Africa. In an uncontrolled study, 48 patients received the tea for four days (5g dried leaves infused in one liter of hot water). After the treatment, 92 percent of patients had no detectable parasites in their bloodstream, and there were significant improvements in subjective symptoms in 70 percent of the treated patients. Recent use of Artemisia annua, or more specifically artemisinin, as an anticancer agent has been studied. This development is based on the finding that cancer cells have a much higher concentration of iron than normal cells. (It is thought that artemisinin interacts with iron to generate reactive oxygen species -- free radicals -- which kill the malaria parasite.) Tests on cancer cell lines have established that artemisinin is also selectively toxic to cancer cells, presumably because their higher iron levels result in cytotoxic effects following free radical generation after contact with artemisinin. This is why antioxidant vitamins should be avoided while on the parasite cleanse. The same mechanism holds true in parasites, cancer and Candida/yeast.

Cloves

The clove is a small evergreen tree with a pyramidal trunk that divides into large branches covered with a smooth grayish bark; the leaves are large, entire, oblong, lanceolate (always bright green color), and the plant stand in pairs on short foot-stalks. When bruised, the plant is very fragrant. Clove flowers grow in bunches at the end of the branches. At the start of the rainy season, long greenish buds appear, and from the extremity of these, the corolla comes which is of a lovely rosy peach color. As the corolla fades, the calyx turns yellow, then red. The calyces, with the embryo seed, are at this stage beaten from the tree and when dried are the cloves of commerce. The flowers have a strong refreshing odor. If the seeds are allowed to mature, most of the pungency is lost. Each berry has only one seed. The clove tree usually produces fruit about eight or nine years after planting. The whole tree is highly aromatic. The spice was introduced into Europe from the fourth to the sixth century. The finest cloves come from Molucca and Pemba where the trees grow better than anywhere else, but they are also imported from the East and West Indies, Mauritius, and Brazil.

In commerce the varieties are known by the names of the localities in which they are grown. Formerly, cloves were often adulterated, but as production increased, the price lowered and fraud has decreased. Cloves contain a large amount of essential oil which is much used in medicine. When of good quality, they are fat, oily, and dark brown in color and give out their oil when squeezed with the finger-nail. When pale color and dry, they are of inferior quality and yield little oil. Clove stalks are sometimes imported and are said to be stronger and more pungent even than the cloves. Clove trees absorb an enormous amount of moisture, and if placed near water, their weight is visibly increased after a few hours. Dishonest dealers often make use of this knowledge in their dealings, and the powdered stems are often sold as pure powdered cloves. The most stimulating and carminative of all aromatics, clove is given in powder form or as an infusion for nausea emesis, flatulence, languid indigestion, and dyspepsia and is used chiefly to assist the action of other medicines. The medicinal properties of clove reside in the volatile oil. The oil must be kept in dark bottles in a cool place. If distilled with water, salt must be added to raise the temperature of ebullition, and the same cloves must be distilled over and over again to get their full essence. The oil is frequently adulterated with fixed oil and oil of pimento and copaiba. As a local irritant, clove stimulates peristalsis. It is a strong germicide, a powerful antiseptic, a feeble local anesthetic applied to decayed teeth, and has been used with success as a stimulating expectorant in phthisis and bronchial troubles. Fresh infusion of cloves contains astringent matter as well as the volatile oil. The infusion and clove water are good vehicles for alkali's and aromatics. Cloves have been reputed by researcher Hulda Clark PhD, as being highly effective in killing the larva or egg stage of the parasite. For parasite cleansing, it is necessary to use fresh cloves that have not been irradiated. Most spices are irradiated with 35,000 times the amount of radiation permitted in a chest x-ray. This is ostensibly done to eradicate bacteria, but spices are generally excellent bactericides, so the irradiation is merely a way of destroying the precious properties of spices. Non-irradiated spices are available from most high-end health foods stores, and we, of course, carry these spices.

Cloves are among the most antibacterial spices known, but as we all know, a few cloves go a long way. Those with some familiarity with herbal medicine know that clove oil is also used to numb pain due to dental infection, but few know that part of the reason clove oil works so well is that it alleviates the infection. Cloves are antiseptic, bactericidal, and antiparasitic. Cloves are among the most potent and volatile of herbs and have been known to melt through their capsules. They have a similar effect on parasite eggs in your body and this is why you will need them. Cloves specifically target all parasite eggs in your body and are used during your program to prevent re-infestation. Cloves contain caryophyllene and tannins which have powerful anti-microbial properties. It is these components thatat actually travel in the bloodstream killing microscopic parasites and all parasitic larvae and eggs. Cloves do not kill the parasites; rather, cloves contain the chemical "eugenol" which melts the hard plastic-like casing around parasite eggs. This allows the larvae inside of the egg to be destroyed. Eugenol is among the most powerful anti-microbial agents known. Eugenol kills all microscopic protozoa and removes parasite eggs in every stage of development. Cloves are tremendously effective in killing malaria, tuberculosis, cholera, scabies and other parasites, viruses, bacteria, and fungi including Candida. Cloves also destroy pseudomonas aeruginosa, all species of shigella, staph and strep.

Diatomaceous Earth

As described earlier in this piece, diatomaceous earth (DE) is fossilized, single celled organisms called diatoms. Diatoms' walls consist of two parts and contain a mineral called silica. Under a very strong microscope, diatoms have very sharp edges.

"DE" has the neat quality of killing insects. (Unfortunately, it kills good ones, like bees and ladybugs, so its use shouldn't be indiscriminate.) DE is 100 percent ecologically safe to the environment and non-poisonous to man and beast. In fact, if you've eaten anything made with flour (like Bisquick), you've eaten DE. DE is a great remover of parasites and intestinal yeasts. It works by physically scraping and by tearing into them outside membrane as if they were being attacked by thousands of tiny knives

DE works by slicing open the exoskeleton (outer, hard covering) of insects, causing them to "bleed" to death. (Actually, their insides leak out, they dehydrate, and die.) This same things happens to yeasts and parasites

When DE is sprinkled on the ground, on an ant mound, or mixed with grains or legumes, it slices and dices the insects that walk through it, but it won't hurt YOU when you ingest it because the 'sharp pieces' are too small to cut you as your membranes are too thick for it to penetrate. (Many farmers deliberately mix DE with animal feed to kill internal parasites in farm animals. The DE in the animal feces even kills the fly maggots that invariably appear in the patties.)

Castor Oil

Castor oil, when encapsulated and frozen, will pass through the stomach and small intestine before dissolving. Freezing the capsule before ingesting totally eliminates the traditional cramping associated with castor oil liquid because the capsules dissolve in the ileum, the last three fifths of the small intestine. Here the digestive tract hydrolyses this oil into recinoleic acid which, while harmless to humans, is deadly to parasites. The ileum connects to the cecum (the lower end of the ascending colon where the large bowel begins) by way of the ileocecal valve, and the majority of parasites of all kinds will nest in the cecum area. This area is warm and moist, providing a plentiful source of fresh food for these poisonous invaders. Castor oil not only suffocates parasites, but it is also nature's penetrating oil for colon plaque. When the castor oil capsule is frozen, it does not act as a laxative, is odorless, and will not "burp" back. Suggested dosage is two to six capsules every 12 hours.

So there you have it, these are the most important items in parasite elimination. When used correctly they are effective in restoring a normal balance to the intestinal tract and eliminate the "Merchants of Mayhem!"

Chapter 12

Common Digestive Complaints

CONSTIPATION

In this chapter, we are going to cover the most stunning material and research probably ever done regarding health care. Some of the conclusions that I will draw may actually stun you; but, nonetheless, they are based on sound authoritative, documented research.

In 1975, a group of British scientists set out to understand and discover why primitive African people had such a low rate of cancer, coronary disease, and -- specifically -- bowel and digestive disease. Their research was quite exhaustive. It covered and included tracking clues that extended all the way back to lunch menus in an African village right through studying bowel habits in an English mill town in 1850. That's quite a variance. These English doctors, working among the native Africans noticed something very peculiar or at least peculiar to them: the native Africans move their bowels somewhere between three to five times a day and, on average, passed well over one pound of fecal material per day. This was a startling contrast compared to the normal English bowel movement of less than four ounces. It is also quite common for the typical English person to move their bowels once a day or even to skip days. Now, we have been taught (unfortunately), by our physicians that moving one's bowels once a day or even every few days is perfectly normal, and for some people it is normal to just move once a week. Analysis of the stools of these primitive African people found the stool to be virtually odorless; to contain the exact amount of friendly bacteria required to keep the digestive system and digestive track healthy and functioning normally; to have very low levels of putrid action and toxic material; and, for the most part, to be far healthier than the average British bowel movement.

Actual investigation into this shows us that the African people have a diet that is very high in fiber. They eat mostly fruits and vegetables that are high in cellulose and other types of fiber like pectins that are particularly high in water content. The water content helps the body pass the fiber through by keeping the bowel and the feces moist. The average African consumes about 24 grams of crude fiber per day compared to about four to six grams found in the typical British or American diet. Upon more in-depth analysis, it was found that the colons of the African people contained very, very low amounts of the toxins and poisonous materials that are normally associated with the bowel.

These toxins and poisonous materials have been directly linked to arthritis, cancer in general and specifically cancer of the bowel, and many other illnesses and diseases. Since these primitive African people had very low amounts of these poisons in their colons, it was concluded this is why they had such a low incidence of bowel cancer, cancer in general, heart disease, arthritis, and many other illnesses.

So, this leads up to our main question. *What is constipation?* Well, at any given time, the digestive track of homo sapiens is able to hold somewhere between three to five meals. That means if you've eaten three to five meals and haven't had a bowel movement, your body is able to cope with that and able to deal with that. Once we go past three to five meals, the colon begins to expand. It can actually expand up to five times its normal size in order to hold more meals that are not being passed. This, however, produces a very bad situation because the longer the food stays in the intestinal track the more apt it is to begin to ferment, putrefy, rot, and act as a breeding ground for bad bacteria, the likes of which can cause different arthritic conditions, immunological problems such as autoimmune illnesses which can be linked to allergies, chemical sensitivities, and different types of rheumatoid arthritis. Parasites and the eggs of parasites can hatch in your intestinal track the longer the food sits there without being passed out into the toilet. Also, as things become more disturbed, a fungus called Candida Albicans is able to start to grow. This intestinal fungus can grow when friendly bacteria are destroyed in your intestinal track. Most common friendly bacteria are destroyed by antibiotic use or by harmful parasites that can get into your food and water. When they get into your intestinal track, these harmful parasites destroy friendly bacteria allowing this fungus called Candida Albicans to grow.

There are over 100 different symptoms possibly caused by this fungus. They range from allergies, asthma, arthritic complaints, digestive complaints, brain fog, fatigue, spaciness, inability to concentrate, skin problems, food reactions: the list goes on and on.

A healthy functioning digestive tract should be able to have a bowel movement in ratio to every meal that is consumed in one given day. Now, this means if someone eats three times a day, they should have three bowel movements. If they eat one time a day, they should have one bowel movement. Simple math will show us that, after one week's time, if someone consumes three meals a day that's 21 meals: Seven days times three meals. If someone has one bowel movement per day, at the end of the week that's one bowel movement times seven days equals seven bowel movements. Where did all the other food go? Most people have been misled into believing that when they have a bowel movement in the morning they are eliminating all the food from the day before. Nothing can be further from the truth. The reason for that is actual analysis and testing show that the average American has a transit time of at least 48 to 72 hours. The word transit is simply referring to transportation time of the feces from the point it enters the mouth to the point it is actually eliminated in the bowel movement. If food is taking 48 to 72 hours to pass through our systems, there is no way that the bowel movement we are having in the morning is eliminating all the meals from the previous day. Now, this can fool you because some foods tend to move through your system faster than others. For instance beets, which can be used as a great marker for this experiment, usually will pass through within 18 to 24 hours. Salads and vegetables and particularly uncooked vegetables and raw fruits tend to move through faster. However, foods of lower fiber content like meats, refined grains and starchier foods tend to move through more slowly, so you may see part of yesterday's meal in your bowel movement and be tricked into thinking that the whole meal was just passed. What actually occurred is some of the foods than can run faster through your digestive tract basically just outran all of the other foods that were there. This doesn't mean the entire meal was passed. On the contrary, it has defiantly been confirmed that it takes 42 to 72 hours for most Americans to pass what we would refer to as the average American meal.

Now, let me ask you this question: How often do you take out your garbage particularly during the summertime? Now, let's look at the garbage for a second. The garbage can has a lid; so, in the garbage can, it is dark and moist, and we have a lot of old food scraps in there. During the summer, if the can is outside, the sun beats on it making it hot, so we have a dark, moist, and warm environment. Now, if you took out your garbage on Monday and then that night filled up the pail again and then left the pail alone until Wednesday or Thursday, what would you expect to smell when you opened up that pail? It certainly wouldn't be anything pleasant or anything to look forward to. Of course not! It would stink. This is because the foods sitting in the garbage pail are mixing with bacteria that were already present in the food and are being allowed to putrefy. I don't think there are that many of us who would expect a garbage pail that has been sitting there for two or three days to be a very healthy environment. So, why would we ever think that our intestinal track would be any healthier if we allow garbage to stay in there for two or three days? A normal healthy person who is eating three meals-a-day should have a bowel movement three times a day or, at minimum, two times if he's eating. If this person who is eating three meals-a-day is not at least two if not three bowel movements each day, the situation that exists is a mild form of constipation.

Now, someone may have bowel movements three or four times-a-day, but if the bowel movements are loose, they won't be passing a lot of solid material and that would still be considered constipation. Remember, constipation means *to compact*; it doesn't mean how many times you are moving. It simply means that things are being compacted in the bowel, and the bowel is not fully evacuating and cleaning itself. Diarrhea in many senses can be a form of severe constipation. If analysis were performed on the bulk weight of the material released in every episode of diarrhea experienced by one person over the period of a few days, the analysis would show that the person passed mostly water and not much solid material. Therefore, the solid material is staying in the bowel; so, even though there seems to be a lot of movement, nothing of value is happening – no cleansing – because the afflicted person is passing water rather than solid material.

Sometimes people can become so constipated that all that will come out is liquid and loose material. This is defiantly a form of constipation if the bowels are being moved every two to three days or any longer than that. This is severe constipation. This is the type of situation that is a breeding ground for many illnesses and diseases. The toxins that are produced in the bowel along with the different microorganisms such as bacteria, parasites, and the fungus Candida Albicans, can produce more symptoms, illnesses, and diseases than anyone can believe.

We have seen arthritis, diabetes, hypoglycemia, muscle soreness and pain, osteoporosis, PMS other reproductive disorders, chronic migraines, and all types of indigestion and digestion complaints clear up miraculously once patients started moving their bowels normally again.

There are many causes of constipation. Very typically, antibiotics and other drugs can disrupt the friendly bacteria called acidophilus and bifidus that live in our intestinal tract. These friendly bacteria help us to digest our food and help keep the intestinal pH at the right balance so that the bowels are able to move. When these bacteria are destroyed, the bowels can become too alkaline. Many times, the stool pH can go over 7.2, which is much more alkaline than it should be. When the stool pH becomes too alkaline, the bowels slow down and constipation is apparent. Different enzymes that help digest food and help us absorb vitamins and minerals stop working. At this point, we are unable to digest and absorb the vitamins, minerals, proteins, and other nutrients from our food, and we start developing many deficiency diseases that many of us read about in health and vitamin books.

Many things can disturb our friendly bacteria. It could be as simple as chlorinated water. Excessive intake of coffee, alcohol, and other drugs can also disturb the friendly bacteria. Friendly bacteria are very commonly disturbed by parasites. This may be horrible to confront and may be very difficult for anyone to want to believe, but people are picking up parasites all the time. We pick up parasites from our pets, from our water, from our food, and even from each other. If the eggs from parasites are allowed to stay in our bodies too long, the eggs come in contact with certain chemicals -- two of them are called propyl alcohol and benzene – and these eggs are allowed to hatch, and then parasites start to grow and multiply in our bodies. Many parasites can lay thousands of eggs a day. Once these parasites start to grow and mature, they disrupt the friendly bacteria, which then can lead, not only to constipation, but also to different parasite symptoms. Many authorities and experts now believe that over 90 percent of all Americans are affected with parasites and that parasites are actually the cause of 50 percent of the ailments and illnesses for which doctors are commonly treating people. Can you imagine that over 50 percent of all the ailments and illnesses for which we are that going to our doctor are actually being caused by parasites living in our bodies as opposed to all these big fancy words and terms that are being coined in medical textbooks?

Constipation can also be caused by nutritional deficiencies that can cause under active adrenal and thyroid function. The adrenal gland acts like the fuel pump in the body helping fuel get into the cells. The thyroid gland acts somewhat like a sparkplug, helping the body burn up fuel and create energy. These two glands also stimulate the digestive system, and it's very common to find constipated people with under active thyroid and adrenal function. Many times, under activity of these glands will not show up on the standard blood test that our doctors will do because this under activity is being caused by mild nutritional deficiencies of the vitamins, minerals, and proteins that help these glands to work. This is when a person needs to see a nutritionist to resolve the matter. Constipation can also be caused by a sluggish liver. This, again, may not show up on standard medical tests because it may not be a disease condition. The liver itself will not stimulate the digestive track to move and pass food along by releasing adequate amounts of bile which is a substance which helps us breakdown fats in our diet. Many experts now feel that almost everyone has gallstones even though they may not be symptomatic or necessarily need medication or surgery from their doctors. Gallstones can start accumulating in the gallbladder in the hundreds and hundreds or even thousands before the person may ever be symptomatic of it. I have seen the proof of this with my own eyes. I have had many patients do something that we call a gallbladder flush. This involves taking some simple every day household foods like lemon and olive oil and some basic herbs that flush the gallstones out of the gallbladder. I have had hundreds of patients do this, and each one has reported seeing hundreds of stones pass, and these were people who were never symptomatic of any type of gallbladder or gallstone problem. What we need to learn from this is that these stones could be in our gallbladder and could be causing the gallbladder and the liver to function ineffectively. This can be another cause of constipation. Constipation might also be caused by certain vitamin or mineral deficiencies including a lack of Pantothenic acid. This is a B vitamin that helps encourage normal peristalsis in the intestines. Peristalsis is the wavelike muscular contraction of the colon in the small intestines that pushes food along, eventually moving it to the end of the colon where it is eliminated out of the body in normal bowel movements.

Probably the three most basic causes of constipation though are much simpler than any one of those mentioned above. The first is lack of water. It's interesting to know that fish do not have colons. The reason for this is that fish are immersed in water all day, and the job of the colon is to reabsorb water from our food so that we can retain the moisture. Mammals and land creatures have colons. They are not immersed in water all the time so, they need to recycle the water from their food in order to avoid dehydration. Many people have had the experience of feeling like they have to have a bowel movement but, for some reason, they aren't able to go when nature was calling. Later, they found the stool was dry and hard to pass. This is because the colon was absorbing excessive amounts of moisture from the stool which then had then become dry. This can happen on a routine basis if there is not enough water in our diet. When an insufficient amount of water is present, fecal matter in the colon will become dry and become stuck in the intestinal tract. These layers of fecal matter can start building up much like rust does on a pipe. The bowel movements that a person like this is having are actually being pushed through these layers of old dried material.

Another cause of constipation is a lack of fiber combined with the consumption of too many junk foods that are low in fiber. Fiber, as we have all learned by now, is essential. It is a bulking material that helps move material along much as a broom brushes material. Nowadays, people are taking Metamucil that is essentially a substance called psyllium. Psyllium is a seed that contains an outer husk that absorbs water and gels and bulks up. When this is consumed, it acts as a fiber laxative. The fiber creates a feeling of fullness and pressure in the colon and stimulates the colon to push fecal matter through thereby also pushing with it the feces that were our food. Foods low in fiber or foods that are commonly thought of as being junk foods cause the intestinal tract to secrete mucus. The mucus is secreted by the intestinal tract as a way of coating itself and protecting itself from these harmful irritating junk foods. Mucus buildup in the colon can also occur from taking drugs, from ingesting too much alcohol, or from having parasites or other harmful organisms in the intestinal tract. Once again, the intestinal tract is only trying to protect itself by secreting mucus in order to put a thin layer of protective fluid between itself and the harmful irritant substance. As time goes on, with the lack of water and fiber in the diet, the low fiber food mixes with the mucus and start to develop into a paste. Eventually it hardens like Plaster of Paris and becomes black and highly toxic. As mentioned earlier, this material can build up like rust in a pipe. It is this material that is literally killing millions and millions of Americans. This material contains many toxic chemical substances, harmful bacteria, parasites, and the fungus Candida Albicans, all of which can be damaging to our health.

A third cause of constipation is insufficient chewing. Chewing helps send signals to our digestive system that food is being consumed. Chewing acts like a stimulus to the digestive system: chewing tells the stomach, pancreas, and the liver to produce digestive juices and tells the intestines and the large bowel to push food along the digestive tract. It is amazing when we realize how much more energy people have when they are able to get rid of these internal poisons that they are carrying around and producing every second from the dirty, toxic bowels that we have in this country.

There is a solution to the problem of constipation: Our new constipation program. This program involves disinfecting the bowel and thereby killing harmful bacteria, fungi, and parasites and their eggs that injure the body and allow constipation to persist. We want to kill these organisms.

The first step in the constipation program is to destroy as many of these organisms as we can so that when we start to clean out the bowel, these bugs don't come up and bite us. If we were to clean out the bowel first, we may end up disturbing the harmful organisms. Imagine what would happen if you disturbed a hornets' nest outside in your backyard. I don't think you want to go over and pick it up and throw it away. I think the first thing you would want to do before you cleaned the hornets' nest out, is throw some bug killer on it to kill as many hornets as you can, so they don't come out and attack you once they find out you're trying to disturb their nest. Well, that's the same concept we have here.

The second step in the constipation program involves the patient actually taking herbal substances and other natural things that help to loosen hardened fecal matter in the colon and then allow it to pass out of the body. Some of the herbs we use are somewhat like jack hammers in how they work; they break up material. Some of the other herbs that are used can be thought of as being more like bulldozers. Once the material has been loosened by the jackhammer, the bulldozer herbs move through and push it out, allowing us to pass it out of the body. At this stage of the constipation program, colonics are sometimes very useful. For those of you who have never heard of this before, a *colonic* is a procedure where a certified technician has you lie down on a table and then inserts a disposable plastic tub into the rectum. The tube that is inserted into your rectum is connected to an apparatus or machinery that allows water to be gradually pumped into the colon and, at the same time, pumps out water that has entered the colon. This creates a flushing action. It is very safe and very gentle, you can think of it as one big continuous enema. The goal of a colonic is never to balloon or overfill your colon causing it to burst; rather, the colonic allows water to gently enter the colon to loosen old fecal matter which is dried and has become stuck in different areas and to flush out this material.

The next step of the constipation program is to help clear the gallbladder and liver of any stones they may have in order to bring these organs up to a more full operating capacity. This step is essential for proper bowel movements. Once the stones are removed, we concentrate on getting friendly bacteria to regrow in the intestinal tract and large bowel. We use very special laboratory-tested strains of human bacteria and other substances that help the friendly bacteria to become established in the colon and large intestine. The result is that the large intestine and colon again have a proper, healthy environment conducive to good digestion and proper bowel movements.

GERD

Gastroesophageal reflux disease (GERD) is a chronic digestive disease that occurs when stomach acid or, occasionally, bile flows back (refluxes) into the food pipe (esophagus). The backwash of acid irritates the lining of the esophagus, mouth, and even sinuses.

The obvious signs and symptoms of GERD include acid reflux and heartburn. Both are common digestive conditions that most people experience from time to time. When these signs and symptoms occur more than twice each week or interfere with daily life, doctors term this GERD. Most people can manage the discomfort of heartburn with lifestyle or diet changes and over-the-counter medications. But, for people with chronic GERD, these remedies may offer only temporary relief. People with chronic GERD may resort to stronger medications that can have harmful side effects: osteoporosis being a common one. Some people have more subtle symptoms of GERD such as chronic sinusitis, running nose, and sore throats.

Signs and Symptoms of GERD

The most-common symptoms of GERD are listed below. A GERD sufferer can have any combination of these:

- Heartburn
- Regurgitations
- Trouble swallowing

Less-common symptoms include

- Pain with swallowing
- Excessive salivation (this is common during heartburn, as saliva is generally slightly basic and is the body's natural response to heartburn, acting similarly to an antacid)
- Nausea
- Chest pain

GERD sometimes causes injury of the esophagus. These injuries may include:

1. Reflux esophagitis causing ulcers near the junction of the stomach and esophagus.
2. Reflux esophagitis causing ulcers near the junction of the stomach and esophagus.
3. Esophageal strictures—the persistent narrowing of the esophagus caused by reflux-induced inflammation.
4. Barrett's esophagus (changes of the epithelial cells from squamous to columnar epithelium) of the distal esophagus.
5. Esophageal adenocarcinoma—a rare form of cancer.

Several other atypical symptoms are associated with GERD, but there is good evidence for causation only when they are accompanied by esophageal injury. These symptoms are:

- Chronic cough
- Laryngitis (hoarseness, throat clearing)
- Asthma
- Erosion of dental enamel
- Sinusitis and damaged teeth

Some people have proposed that symptoms such as pharyngitis, sinusitis, recurrent ear infections, and idiopathic pulmonary fibrosis are due to GERD.

What is GERD?

GERD is not an ulcer; it is a splash back of acid and digestive juices into the throat. It's that simple. The question becomes, "What is causing this to occur."

A simple but important concept to grasp is that if the stomach doesn't produce enough acid to correctly digest food, the food will regurgitate up the throat and cause GERD or as the Italian people call it "Ageda." Food that is not digested well in the stomach will not be allowed to pass from the stomach into the intestines; instead, it will reflux back up the esophagus. This is one of the more common forms of GERD and is due to a lack of stomach acid, not an excess. This will be covered in detail in this article as it is a major cause of GERD which is commonly misunderstood.

H. PYLORI

Years ago, "stress" was thought to be c common cause of for stomach ulcers. Thanks to the work of two Australian doctors -- Robin Warren, M.D., and Barry Marshall, M.D. – who, in the early 1980s discovered the bacterium *Helicobacter Pylori,* we now know that H. Pylori is the primary cause for peptic and duodenal ulcers. Some doctors place the bacterium's involvement as high as 90 percent, but ulcer-inducing drugs, alcohol, and other lifestyle stimulants are still a common factor in the development of ulcers. H. Pylori itself can lower stomach acid which, in turn, causes food to "repeat or reflux" creating the symptoms called GERD.

H. Pylori can be inhibited by increasing the amount of stomach acid; so, if a person with H. Pylori drinks Apple Cider Vinegar (ACV), the ACV will inhibit the H. Pylori allowing for an increase in stomach acid and for more complete digestion thereby lessening the GERD.

Unfortunately, people with *reduced acid levels* frequently suffer from what they *assume is elevated stomach acid* (heartburn, bloating, nausea, frequent burping) and subsequently take acid-lowering drugs or remedies. This can temporarily improve the symptoms of GERD because the stomach contains a sensor that allows food to leave and pass into the small intestines when it detects that the stomach acid levels are declining. The body would like to believe the levels are declining because the stomachs digestive process is completed. But, the stomach can be tricked into thinking the digestive process is complete by the introduction of antacids. The use of antacids actually encourages greater H. Pylori activity and thus increases the risk of developing peptic or duodenal ulcers, pancreatic / gastric cancer, and mucosa-associated lymphoid tissue (MALT) lymphoma.

GERD AND H. PYLORI

About 60 percent of all the GERD patients I have seen have H. Pylori. It is controversial in mainstream medicine as to whether or not H. Pylori causes GERD. The confusion usually stems from two factors:

1. The testing used to determine H. Pylori is often inaccurate. The test I favor is a stool test called the GI EFFECTS TEST. This test looks for DNA of H. Pylori as well as other microorganisms that can cause

GERD. This test is the most accurate way I know of to detect H. Pylori.

2. The 2nd factor is that esophageal reflux (GERD) can be caused by a lack of stomach acid, not excess stomach acid. Because it is assumed that GERD must be from excess acid, not from inadequate acid caused by the presence of H. Pylori, testing is often omitted. After the discovery of Helicobacter Pylori, and once medical science accepted H. Pylori as being a significant factor with ulcers, predictions were made that ulcers and related stomach complaints would become a thing of the past. However, there are as many patients as ever complaining of stomach problems, including those who had been "cured" of H. Pylori. The reason for is very simply that low stomach acid has not been corrected as part of the treatment. As a self-test, if the consumption of HCL tablets or Apple Cider Vinegar worsens the symptoms of GERD, there is a significant possibility that H.Pylori is not and never was the underlying cause of GERD. However, this is not fool proof!

The Problem of Testing for H. Pylori

Physicians don't generally test for Helicobacter Pylori unless a patient exhibits gastric complaints and, even if a patient suffers from non-gastric symptoms, there is little chance of the average practitioner relating any of the symptoms. Patients frequently have to convince or even *beg* their GPs to run a test after the patient learns about H. Pylori through a news flash or from reading about the long-term risks associated with its infection. Unfortunately, testing can also be inaccurate. Blood antibody tests that are often preferred can give false negatives as can gastric biopsies.

I prefer the GI EFFECTS STOOL TEST. This is a test that looks for DNA of various harmful micro-organisms. The key problem I have found is that doctors testing for H. Pylori will not find it even though it is present, so they can't correlate its presence to GERD or to other digestive maladies.

When using blood tests for H. Pylori, it is not uncommon that the blood remains positive for H. Pylori for up to nine months after the infection is cleared. This also makes the correlation of H. Pylori difficult with testing and treatments. The lack of effective testing to properly identify H. Pylori has resulted in flawed research and conclusions relative to how common H. Pylori can be in GERD- related disorders.

The Different Types of Cases

Low Acid Case It is very important to understand the cause of each patient's GERD rather than simply suppressing the symptoms. In many cases, patients with GERD actually have low stomach acid and not excess stomach acid as explained earlier. In these cases, the low stomach acid causes food to be improperly digested, so it is regurgitated and therefore causes GERD. These patients may have H. Pylori which decreases stomach acid as well as a Hiatal Hernia which then entraps the acid.

High Acid Case The other type of case occurs when the patient actually does produce excess stomach acid. This can be due to stress or any condition that causes the "sympathetic nervous system" to become excessively stimulated. This can occur in the "Type-A" personality who is on the go and under a lot of stress. High Acid patients may also consume substances like coffee, tobacco, herbal stimulants, and drugs that are stimulating and may further increase their stomach acid. Excessively high Adrenal, Thyroid, or Pancreatic function can be a cause. Gallstones which block or congest the Gallbladder can also be a cause.

Candida, Parasites & GERD

Other microorganism such as Candida, protozoa (parasites), and bacteria can also cause reflux. I have been quite surprised over the years by observing just how many of our Candida patients have had their GERD resolve as the Candida was eliminated. Many protozoa (microscopic parasites) such as amoebas, giardia, and entamoeba can cause GERD; however, other symptoms such as nausea, loss of appetite, and an upper gastro-intestinal uneasiness will normally accompany the GERD. These signs are often followed by or accompanied by a sudden onset of explosive, watery, foul-smelling diarrhea. Stools associated with giardia infection are generally described as loose, bulky, frothy, and/or greasy with the absence of blood or mucus. Other gastro-intestinal disturbances associated with giardiasis include flatulence, bloating, anorexia, cramps, and foul sulfuric belching (sometimes called 'purple burbs').

So these are the two basic types of GERD: that caused by too little acid and that caused by too much. The other condition that can cause GERD is structural. By *structural* I am referring to a mechanical imbalance in the alignment of the spine or a problem with the valves that lead from the esophagus to stomach, stomach to small intestines, small intestines to colon etc. The valves can become sluggish and can remain partially opened or closed which allows the GERD. The valve problems listed below can cause bile produced by the liver to flow unchecked into the small intestine which then triggers partially digested food in the upper part of the small intestine and the stomach to reflux up the esophagus and cause "GERD."

1. Hiatal Hernia.
2. Ileocecal Valve
3. Houstons Valve

Very often reflux or GERD can occur due to structural problems that can cause either a Hiatal Hernia that can entrap acids, the improper function of the valves in the intestinal tract, or specific spinal misalignments that can cause improper nerve flow to the digestive organs. A chiropractor who understands these concepts and who is skilled in correcting them will actually realign these area and get the structure back into balance.

Many chiropractors specialize in "Ileocecal Valve" problems. Ileocecal valve problems that can lead to reflux and other digestive problems.

Could It Be Your Ileocecal Valve?

The Ileocecal valve is often an underlying cause of GERD that will go completely ignored unless the patient is lucky enough to visit a practitioner who is familiar with its function – or dysfunction as the case may be. The Ileocecal Valve is located between the ileum (last portion of your small intestine) and the cecum or ascending colon (first portion of your large intestine), and the appendix lies just below it. The function of the ileocecal valve is to allow digested food materials to pass from the small intestine into the large intestine. The ileocecal valve also blocks these waste materials from backing up into the small intestine. It is intended to be a one-way valve, only opening up to allow the digested material to pass through and then closing to prevent the fecal contents from "falling" back into the small intestine. When the small intestine/large intestine is not active in the process of digestion or stool production), the value is relaxed, neither open nor closed.

Ileocecal Valve Syndrome

When the ileocecal valve is stuck open, waste products can back up into the small intestine (much like a backed up kitchen sink drain) disturbing the digestion and also creating unhealthy toxins that are absorbed into the body. Also, if the ileocecal valve is stuck closed, waste products are prevented or constricted from passing into the large intestine. Either way, the end result can be GERD. Unfortunately, this disorder is often overlooked by the medical profession. A dysfunctional ileocecal valve can result in a combination of symptoms. Ileocecal valve problems can very often produce GERD.

Ileocecal Valve Syndrome Signs & Symptoms:

- Dark circles under eyes

- Bowel disturbances (diarrhea / constipation)
- Weakness of the Psoas, Iliacus, or Quadriceps muscles – muscles involved in posture and locomotion
- Low back pain – esp. pain on bending over
- Severe lumbar disc complaints (sharp, sudden pain)
- Sinus problems, post nasal drip, headaches, tinnitus
- GERD symptoms
- Joint pains
- Pelvic congestion and pain
- PMS
- Chronic inflammatory or toxicity complaints

Self Help Treatments

Until a person can get properly tested to determine the true underlying cause of your GERD, the following self-treatments can serve:

1. To help the symptoms, or until any of several possible causes for low stomach acid or high acid are resolved, a digestive aid containing Glutamic acid + Betaine + Pepsin should be taken with every larger meal. Some patients also have good results using Lemon or Lime Water. The only contraindications are gastritis, the presence of an ulcer, or high stomach acid levels are high that would prohibit the use of acid-raising supplements.
2. Bromelain, known for its anti-inflammatory and digestive support, may be another consideration to help a low stomach acid environment – with or without reflux, but particularly when reflux is present, provided there are no contraindications to bromelain's mild blood-thinning properties.
3. When antibiotics and natural approaches have not been successful in eradicating H. Pylori, or when there is intolerance to most of the remedies that are usually helpful with low-acid symptoms, then regularly drinking Pineapple Juice with meals or

sipping it slowly throughout the day is another option that has helped many patients reduce their symptoms and improve general digestion.

4. Maintain a healthy weight. Excess pounds put pressure on the abdomen, pushing up the stomach and causing acid to back up into the esophagus. If your weight is healthy, work to maintain it. If you are overweight or obese, work to slowly lose weight — no more than 1 or 2 pounds (0.5 to 1 kilogram) a week. Ask your doctor for help devising a weight loss strategy that will work for you.
5. Avoid tight-fitting clothing. Clothes that fit tightly around your waist put pressure on your abdomen and lower esophageal sphincter.
6. Avoid foods that trigger heartburn. Everyone has specific triggers. Common triggers such as fatty or fried foods, alcohol, chocolate, mint, garlic, onion, and caffeine may make heartburn worse.
7. Don't lie down after a meal. Wait at least two to three hours after eating before lying down or going to bed.
8. Elevate the head of your bed. An elevation of about six to nine inches puts gravity to work for you. Place wood or cement blocks under the feet of your bed at the head end. If it's not possible to elevate your bed, insert a wedge between your mattress and box spring to elevate your body from the waist up. Wedges are available at drugstores and medical supply stores.
9. Don't smoke. Smoking decreases the lower esophageal sphincter's ability to function properly.

Suffer from food allergies and sensitivities? Consider "Leaky Gut"

Leaky Gut is a very common condition in this day and age. It is the cause of much or our modern autoimmune illness, IBS, Crohn's disease, allergies, asthma, food sensitivities, chemical sensitivities, arthritic conditions, etc. It is an illness that depicts our modern times.

A gut that has become inflamed will become very porous (much more porous than it should be) which will allow large food proteins, bacteria, fungi, metals, and toxic substances straight into the blood stream. This is the basis of "Leaky Gut Syndrome." In more scientific language, an increase in permeability of the intestinal mucosa to luminal macromolecules, antigens, and toxins associated with inflammatory degenerative and/or atrophic mucosal damage. Once in the blood stream, our immune system is the last line of defense to deal with these substances, and it will eventually get overwhelmed if a Leaky Gut is not rectified.

Cause of Leaky Gut Syndrome

Our intestinal lining replaces itself approximately every 24 hours. This means that every cell of which the lining is composed is digested or sloughed off, and a new one grows to take its place. All this activity means the gut uses more blood when it is resting than any other organ, but it is also the first to lose its blood supply when in a fight-or- flight situation, which is what stress is. If you have a lot of stress, then your gut will always be starved for blood and the lining will be impaired.

The key and most common cause of Leaky Gut is Candida. Candida is a yeast-fungal organism that grows roots like a plant. These roots grow into and through your intestinal tract looking for food. These roots break through the intestinal lining and cause the leaky gut!

The Big Confusion

Leaky gut causes many of the severe symptoms of Candida. Removing Candida can often help Leaky Gut but removing Candida often does not heal the Leaky Gut unto itself. After Candida is gone, Leaky Gut is still there and so are the Leaky Gut symptoms. So the person may think

Candida is still present, but it's not! And if the person and the doctor continue to treat the Candida, they will see no improvement because what they should be treating is the Leaky Gut!

Acidophilus Makes me Sick!

People with Leaky Gut lose their *Mucin layer.* Mucins protect the intestinal cells and act like a barrier similar to wax on your car or wood floor. When the Mucin layer is gone due to Leaky Gut, you may react allergically to Acidophilus. If Acidophilus makes you bloat, have gas, itch, or gives you rashes, hives, flu symptoms, and allergy reactions you may have Leaky Gut Syndrome.

Other factors that cause or worsen Leaky Gut Syndrome are:

1. Alcohol and caffeine which irritate the gut wall, this includes cola drinks (diet and regular), chocolate, coffee, and cocoa.
2. Contaminated foods. E. coli and other bacteria's can develop due to poor food handling.
3. Chemicals found in processed and fermented foods (dyes and preservatives),wine, vinegar, soy sauce, tofu, etc.
4. A diet high in refined sugars and other carbohydrates (e.g. candy, cookies, sodas, processed foods and white bread).
5. Foods contaminated by parasites (pork, chicken, fresh water and hatchery fish).
6. Antibiotic use. This causes an overgrowth of fungi (yeast) in the gut due to the immune suppression that occurs.
7. Ingestion of animal products that have been given hormonal and antibiotic treatments.
8. NSAIDs (non-steroidal anti-inflammatory drugs).

The Mucous System's Role

The mucous system in our nasal passages flushes bacteria and viral particles into our stomach where the hydrochloric acid (HCL) should kill them. Any that get through to a normal gut should eventually be excreted. Of course, a Leaky Gut will let bacteria and viral particles into the bloodstream. When leaky gut is improved, a great number of harmful organisms are kept out of the body. These include:

- Air-borne allergy-causing contaminants such as household dust (mite feces) and pollens are kept from entering the tissue of the lungs and nasal passages, thus reducing the effects of hay fever and asthma.
- Industrial contaminants such as exhaust gasses, solvents etc. are also kept at bay.
- Parasites such as Cryptosporidium, giardia, salmonella, even hookworm can be dissuaded from entering the walls of the stomach and intestines. This coating can also provide a hostile living environment for parasites.
- The mucus provides a shield that prevents the roots of the Candida yeast culture from penetrating the intestine wall, thus reducing the severity of this disease.
- Undigested food and toxins are deterred from entering the blood stream thus reducing one of the most common causes of allergies and autoimmune diseases.

The 7 Stages of the 'Inflamed' Gut

1. When the gut is inflamed, it does not absorb nutrients and foods properly and so fatigue and bloating can occur.
2. As mentioned previously, when large food particles are absorbed, there is the creation of food allergies and new symptoms with target organs, such as arthritis or fibromyalgia.
3. When the gut is inflamed, the carrier proteins are damaged so nutrient deficiencies occur that can also cause many symptoms like magnesium deficiency induced muscle spasm or copper deficiency induced high cholesterol.
4. Likewise, when the detox pathways that line the gut are

compromised, chemical sensitivity can arise. Furthermore the leakage of toxins overburdens the liver so that the body is less able to handle everyday chemicals.

5. When the gut lining is inflamed, the protective coating of the IgA (immunoglobulin A) is adversely affected and the body is not able to ward off protozoa, bacteria, viruses, and yeast's like Candida. When the intestinal lining is inflamed, bacteria and yeast's are able to translocate. This means that they are able to pass from the gut lumen or cavity, into the bloodstream and set up infection anywhere else in the body.
6. The worst symptom is the formation of antibodies. Sometimes these leak across and look similar to antigens on our own tissues. Consequently, when an antibody is made to attack it, it also attacks our tissue. This is probably how autoimmune disease start. Rheumatoid arthritis, lupus, multiple sclerosis, thyroiditis, and many others are members of this ever-growing category of 'incurable' diseases.

Diseases Caused By Leaky Gut Syndrome

- Chronic Fatigue Syndrome
- Rheumatoid Arthritis
- Asthma
- Multiple Sclerosis
- Fibromyalgia
- Vasculitis
- Crohn's Disease
- Addison's Disease
- Lupus
- Thyroiditis

Another problem a leaky gut creates is a mineral deficiency because the inflammatory process damages carrier proteins that are needed for the transport of specific minerals. For example, a magnesium deficiency is present in most Fibromyalgia patients.

The patient can take incredibly high doses of magnesium, but if the carrier protein for this mineral is damaged, no matter how much of the mineral the patient takes, the mineral will not get into the body where it is needed. This can also be true for some bone disorders. A zinc deficiency will affect hair loss and some eye disorders (macular degeneration). Copper deficiency can also occur this way and can lead to Osteoarthritis or even elevated blood cholesterol in some cases. If you have any syndrome that could be connected to a mineral deficiency, or if you exhibit symptoms that don't seem to go away no matter what you do, you should consider the possibility of a leaky gut.

Healing A Leaky Gut

In order to heal Leaky Gut we must first disinfect the intestines of all the infections we can cause or prevent the gut from healing. In 1990, I began to describe the new approach to Candida. The new approach first eliminated parasites and the top layers of Candida and used natural killers to destroy the Candida throughout the body. The killers are taken on a four-day rotation so that the Candida will not become immune to them. The next step is to destroy the Candida deep in the lining of intestines where it will cause Leaky Gut. Once this is done, the leaky gut can be healed using the Leaky Gut Protocol. There are many products made today for leaky gut syndrome. Most contain Glutamine, MSM, zinc, essential fatty acids, intestinal protein concentrate, white fish proteins, Mucins, and vitamins and minerals that help to reduce inflammation and heal the gut lining. After Leaky Gut is healed you can then take and benefit from acidophilus.

The Leaky Gut Testing

In order to determine which product will the best and the length of time needed on the products, we perform a Leaky Gut test. The intestinal permeability test is performed in the following way. A solution of two non-metabolizable sugars is consumed. One of these sugars is normally absorbed by the intestinal mucosa, the other is not. Urine is collected for several hours after drinking the solution, and a sample is sent to the laboratory for analysis. When the normally non-absorbed sugar is found at high concentration in the urine, this indicates Leaky Gut Syndrome. If the normally absorbed sugar is found to be lacking in the urine, this is a sign of malabsorption. Results of the intestinal permeability test lead to appropriate follow-up evaluation and natural therapies to restore normal permeability.

It seems that in most people who are chemically sensitive or allergic to anything, the very first flaw in their system is that their intestinal tract is lacking a protective coating, or worse yet, has *intestinal permeability* (which is also called "leaky gut syndrome"). When someone lacks the protective coating in their intestinal tract, foods, chemicals, and microorganisms such as parasites, bacteria, and viruses can begin irritating the lining of the intestinal tract. What will happen next is that the immune system will start reacting at the line of the intestinal tract in order to fight back. This creates inflammation, swelling, and further irritation of the intestinal lining. Beside causing intestinal pain, intestinal cramps, and irritation, this will begin allergic reactions throughout the body. It seems that these allergic reactions, begun in the intestinal tract, trigger skin reactions such as itching, hives, and rashes. As this continues for a length of time, the next step is that the intestinal lining becomes further degraded and starts to actually develop barriers that are leaky. The normal villi in the intestinal tract, (hair-like structures that help absorb vitamins, minerals, and different nutrients from your food) become damaged. These tiny hairs are not able to absorb the nutrients from your food that are passing through your intestines and so are unable to send the nutrients into your bloodstream so your cells, glands and organs can use them.

Instead, holes -- or leaky patches -- develop at different points in the intestinal tract. These holes allow large particles of foods, pollens, chemicals, microorganisms, and other harmful detritus fall between the cracks and into your bloodstream. If these holes or leaks were not present, these harmful substances would never be able to get into your bloodstream. However, once these harmful factors are in your bloodstream, they create havoc: bad reactions and environmental allergies result. This is how the person then becomes an "allergic to everything" type of person.

One of the major differences between someone who is HIV positive and someone who has full-blown AIDS is that the person with full-blown AIDS has developed this leaky gut syndrome. Naturally, due to that, the AIDS patient is much more susceptible to contracting other infections and other problems. The person who is merely HIV positive -- who doesn't have this leaky gut syndrome -- has more protection because the intestinal tract is not allowing harmful organisms to pass through. It is correct to say that, most likely, all people suffering from any type of skin rash or sensitivity have, to some degree, this syndrome of leaky gut or a weakened protective lining of the intestinal tract.

The good news is that this situation can be remedied. Using some of the substances I mentioned earlier -- the plant substances called *mucins* -- to rebuild the friendly protective coating of the intestinal tract and then using other specific nutrients that have been found to be able to rebuild the actual lining of the intestinal tract itself and to strengthen it so as to repair the leaky patches, this problem can be resolved in a matter of a few months.

The first step in handling this problem is to ascertain exactly what's happening in the person's digestive system. A new test has been developed to enable a practitioner to determine the total amount of friendly and harmful bacteria and the amounts of yeast and parasites in a person's intestines, to indicate whether or not the patient is missing the substances in the intestines that protect the lining of the intestines, and to indicate whether or not the intestinal tract has become leaky.

This test also scans the digestive system and the absorption system to see if the patient is digesting and absorbing everything correctly from their food. Furthermore, the test also tells a great deal about how well the immune system is functioning in the intestinal tract. This is the ideally suited test to determine exactly what treatment is needed by someone suffering from this syndrome.

After the testing, the first is to put the person on a program to clear out any harmful bacteria or harmful microorganisms that are living in the intestines. Once they're eliminated, we then can begin building up the friendly bacteria in the system, and then we can begin repairing the intestinal tract.

In some cases, even though harmful organisms are present in the intestines and could continue to break down the intestinal tract causing the same problem all over again, it is necessary to strengthen and heal the intestinal tract a bit before we begin to clear away these harmful organisms. This is true in cases where people are so chemically sensitive or so allergic that they can no longer even tolerate taking the natural substances that might be able to clear away the harmful bacteria or microorganisms from their system. If this is the case, the person first needs a round or so of these substances to strengthen the intestinal tract so that the patient is able to tolerate the substances that remove the harmful bacteria and/or harmful parasites.

Once the intestinal track is strengthened, the person is able to tolerate friendly bacteria. So, those who are very, very sensitive have to actually begin the entire program by correcting as best as we can the weakness of the intestinal lining that causes the bad reaction before beginning the program to totally and completely correct the problem.

This is permissible because after treatment has cleared away the bad microorganisms and then starts to establish friendly bacteria, the patient can then go back on the substances that heal the intestinal tract for a longer period of time so as to obtain a complete and thorough regeneration of the area.

Chapter 13

Mycobacteria

The Greek "myco" refers to fungi or yeast. The manner in which Mycobacteria form and grow on a culture medium (the disk used to grow bacteria in a lab) has earned them this name because they resemble a creature that is half yeast and half bacteria. Think about those horror movies that have monsters that are half man and half animal: Mycobacteria are like that!

Just as was the case with Candida 20 years ago, mainstream medicine is clueless as in how to kill these infections. However, mainstream medicine is more aware of the existence of these infections then they were of Candida 20 years ago. It is my opinion that these infections are caused when bacteria and fungus mutate to live together in a colony or a commune where they cooperate as two distinct organisms and each benefits from the survival of the other as a group and as a single self-protected entity.

Mycobacterium is its own family, the *Mycobacteriaceae*. The family includes pathogens known to cause serious diseases in mammals including tuberculosis and leprosy. The *myco* means "fungus," alluding to the way mycobacteria have been observed to grow in a mold-like fashion on the surface of cultures. Routine antibacterial treatment for bacteria and fungus do not help eliminate these pathogens. There are several thousands of types of Mycobacteria, they affect the lungs, heart, kidneys and urinary tract, intestinal tract, and lymph nodes.

The digestive track is a system vulnerable to infection by atypical bacteria such as mycoplasma and mycobacterium through ingestion. Mycobacteria are commonly found in soil, water and food. It has been thought that they do not cause illness in healthy people and only affect people who have compromised immune system such as AIDS patients. This however is false! Due to new better detection methods, mycobacterial infection has been found in immunocompetent individuals. Individuals can become infected when their immune system is weakened due to stress, aging, or other acute or chronic infections. Young children whose immune system has not fully matured are especially vulnerable. The digestive tract is one of the most commonly infected systems.

Here are some interesting points about these organisms:

1) There are several thousand types.
2) 80 percent of the human population carry these.
3) They are resistant to common drug treatments.
4) Unfortunately they also can be resistant to botanical and herbal treatments if these treatments aren't properly administered.
5) They remain very resistive pathogens even after extensive treatment.
6) They cause autoimmune illnesses of all kinds.
7) They cause allergy symptoms of all kinds by sensitizing the immune system.
8) They cause COPD lung degeneration by damaging lung tissue.
9) They cause sarcoidosis.
10) They suppress the immune system.
11) They inhibit connective tissue growth. Patients with these infections can develop muscle tendon joint and bone pain.
12) They can infect other organs such as the stomach, kidneys, liver, lung, heart, and spleen.
13) They typically cause chronic pneumonia. As the infected lung cells die off, they leave behind fluid filled cysts.
14) They tend to group themselves in a bundle and then secrete a slime coating that protects them against the immune system's

attack and against medicines whether prescription or over-the-counter.

15) The only way they can be killed is to first cut through the slime secretion that they make to protect themselves, thereby allowing the medicines that you take to be able to penetrate their bundles and kill the infection within. How to do this is the trick.

If you have been battling chronic reoccurring infections, regardless of the kind of infection or the area of the body infected for the past several years, odds are you are dealing with MYCOBACTERIA.

Mycobacterium in the digestive tract produce "biofilms" which are a slime that covers the bacteria or fungal cell and protects it from attack by the immune system and from medicines all of kinds: herbal, pharmaceutical etc.

In many cases, these biofilms are the reason some people don't respond to treatments correctly.

After studying the cases of patients who had disappointing results from our program and from the programs of other friendly practices, I have discovered that "Biofilms" may be the missing link that prevents treatments from working correctly. Unlike free-floating bacteria that drift in fluids, biofilms consist of bacteria/fungi that settle onto surfaces and begin to form large clumps surrounded by a protective coating of slime. Biofilms are different from so-called superbugs like MRSA that are resistive to antibiotics. Each individual bacterium in a biofilm would, on its own, be susceptible to modern drugs, but when they clump together, the bacteria morph into complex 3-D structures. Using a vocabulary of chemicals, the bacteria in the biofilms self-organize and divide up tasks. Some grow and secret slime, some dispersing to colonize new areas, and some hibernate until they are needed. The biofilm structures even contain channels to take in nutrients and expel waste. They communicate with each other and coordinate their activity. In a biofilm, you see the cooperative behavior of pathogens, which are disease producing organisms.

Why are Biofilm So Difficult to Kill?

First, there's the slime that antibiotics and herbals have difficulty penetrating. In addition, electrical charges on the slime's surface can form a barrier that keeps out antibiotics. Because many cells deep within a biofilm are nutrient and oxygen starved, they grow fairly slowly and are therefore less susceptible to antibiotics which work best on actively dividing cells. To make matters worse, biofilms contain zombie-like cells which lie dormant when antibiotics are present but spring into action after antibiotic treatment ends. Finally, cells within biofilms can organize themselves to pump drugs right out of cells.

Past Solutions

In the past, we relied upon Biamin, a standard product on our first step of treatment to kill and eliminate biofilm. We have now discovered that biofilm has become more and more aggressive due to antibiotic use, and the use of Biaminis not enough to handle biofilm. Wei Labs, a California based laboratory that creates unique Chinese herbal medicines has now developed a line of herbals that eliminate biofilms and their underlying infections called Mycobacterium.

Mycobacteria avium complex (MAC) is one of the most common mycobacteria that infect the digestive tract. MAC consists of two species: M avium and M intracellulare. Mycobacterium avium, subspecies paratuberculosis (MAP), a closely related subspecies of MAC, can also invade the digestive tract. They are found in many places including tap water, fresh and ocean water, milk, bird droppings, soil, and house dust.

Mycobacteria tuberculosis is an airborne pathogen that mainly infects lungs and causes TB with lung structure damage. Research results have suggested that M. tuberculosis can also cause digestive tract infections because the infected macrophage can carry the bacteria to the digestive system through blood circulation. Each year, tuberculosis (TB) results in the death of three million people globally. If controls are not taken, between the years 2000-2020, an estimated one billion people will be infected, 200 million people will become sick, and 35 million will die from TB.

Multiple strains of Mycoplasma can infect the digestive tract including Mycoplasma pneumoniae, Mycoplasma incognitus, Mycoplasma penetrans, Mycoplasma genitalium, and Mycoplasma hominis. Mycoplasma pneumonia is a common respiratory pathogen that produces respiratory diseases ranging from upper respiratory tract infection to atypical pneumonia. Many patients infected with M. pneumoniae may experience extra pulmonary complications after the onset of or even in the absence of respiratory illness and symptoms.

Gastrointestinal manifestations are frequent and have been described in roughly 25 percent of cases with the acute manifestation of nausea, vomiting, and loss of appetite.

Toxicities

Mycobacterium avium, subspecies paratuberculosis and Inflammatory Bowel Disease Mycobacterium avium, subspecies paratuberculosis (MAP) has been consistently identified in biopsies of the intestinal lining of Crohn's disease patients. Research results also suggest that ulcerative colitis is also caused by MAP. Research on several groups of patients found that for a given age, a small dose of MAP causes ulcerative colitis, while a large dose of MAP causes Crohn's disease. When infected with a small dose of MAP, adults develop ulcerative colitis relatively soon after being infected, while children develop Crohn's disease after a long latency period.

Crohn's disease and ulcerative colitis are chronic gastrointestinal tract diseases that together are referred to as idiopathic inflammatory bowel disease (IIBD), a disease commonly viewed as an autoimmune condition. Although the mechanism how this gram-positive intracellular pathogen triggers autoimmunity is not fully understood, MAP has been viewed as the common culprit for both Crohn's disease and ulcerative colitis. Infection of the MAP causes a chronic intestinal immune inflammatory response, which results in intestinal ulcerations. In ulcerative colitis, only the lining of the colon is affected. The lining of the colon becomes inflamed and develops tiny open sores, or ulcers, that produce pus and mucous. Crohn's disease can affect any part of the gastrointestinal (GI) tract from the mouth to the anus and all layers of the bowel wall. In Crohn's disease, the deep tissues that are affected can form fistulas, abnormal connections between organs. Common symptoms of Crohn's disease and ulcerative colitis are persistent diarrhea accompanied by abdominal pain and blood in the stool, vomiting, severe pelvic pain, and weight loss. MAP can also affect the liver and cause hepatitis.

Humans can get the MAP infection through consumption of contaminated milk, products made from contaminated milk, or via contaminated water caused by feces from infected cattle, cows, pigs, and other domestic animals. MAP is more robust than tuberculosis, and therefore the risk conveyed to human populations in retail milk and domestic water supplies is high. MAP is harbored in the ileocolonic mucosa of a proportion of normal people and can be detected in a high proportion of full thickness samples of inflamed Crohn's disease gut samples.

Diagnosis of MAP infection is difficult. It grows extremely slow. Even when present in immense quantities, it can take several months to even detect MAP in the clinical setting.

Food Allergies, Stomach/Intestinal Ulcer, and Leaky Gut
Mycoplasma pneumoniae is a mucosal pathogen. Its pathogenesis begins with attachment to the surface of epithelial cells followed by release of toxins such as peroxide and superoxide. The attachment induces infiltration of lymphocytes and plasma cells and induces production of multiple arrays of cytokines. These cytokines and toxins cause inflammation and injury to the epithelial tissue structure. Mycoplasma can also fuse its cell membrane with the epithelial cell and become an intracellular organism and further replicate inside the epithelial cells.

The Mycoplasma steals lipids and cholesterol from the mitochondria. This makes the mitochondria 'leaky,' and they lose electrons thus causing reduced efficiency in ATP production. As the mycoplasma adopts host cellular components to replicate, their cell membrane structure begins to mimic the host cell surface composition, causing autoimmunity since the immune system cannot differentiate the mycoplasma from the host's own cells. The infection can cause cell death. After the infected cell dies, the replicated bacteria are released and infect nearby healthy cells. As more infected cells die, a fluid filled cyst will form on the mucosal membrane.

Mycoplasma infection of digestive tract mucosal membranes can destroy intestinal villi and compromise the intestinal barrier. This allows accelerated damage by lectins in grains (especially wheat), beans, soy, and dairy leading to ulcer formation and leaky guts with increased permeability of the mucosal membrane. Patients may experience symptoms such as food sensitivities, gluten intolerance, abdominal pain/cramps, constipation and/or diarrhea, nutritional deficiency and weight loss. The infection can cause significantly increase of the proportion of CD4+ and CD8+ T cells that secreted IL-4, and elevated IgE levels which associates with a Th1/Th2 cytokine imbalance. Such disruption to the intestinal immune system can cause an imbalance of gut flora, over growth of unfriendly germs, and infection of the digestive tract by other types of pathogens including gram-positive bacteria, gram-negative bacteria, fungi, H. Pylori, gram-negative spirochete, protozoa, and many types of parasites. Chronic infection can cause intestinal degenerative changes that allow the microbes to penetrate the intestine and get to the peritoneal spaces and cause pain or discomfort in the lower abdomen.

Infection of gastric mucosa and stomach lining together with the coinfection of other types of microbes can cause chronic gastritis with nausea and stomach discomfort as well as stomach ulcers, intestinal inflammation, and ulcerative changes. Patients may experience stomach and/or abdominal pain/cramping, gas, bloating, acid reflux, diarrhea and constipations.

Digestive Tract Cancers

Intracellular Mycobacterial infection can interrupt the regular programed cell death process causing polyp growth. The infection can also make its way into the nucleus and disrupt the host genome causing malignant transformations. Types of cancer associated with Mycoplasma include colon cancer, gastric cancer, lung cancer, prostate cancer, and renal cancer. Using immunohistochemistry assay and nested polymerase-chain reaction (PCR), researchers have successfully detected Mycoplasma hyorhinis and Mycoplasma fermentans in gastric cancer tissues and found the correlation between mycoplasma infection and characteristics for gastric cancer patients.

How do You Know if You Have Mycobacteria?

The following is the simplest criteria to determine the presence of mycobacteria.

First, confirm you have Candida. Simply observing reactions to high carbs and sugar does this. Does this cause asthma, rashes, inflammation of any kind, bloating, gas, diarrhea or constipation, fatigue, or mental fogginess? If you react adversely to sugar in this manner there is a strong chance you have Candida.

Secondly, do you have a poor treatment history regarding Candida? Does it appear that treatments do not work at all or rollercoaster? Have you failed to obtain stable results from Candida treatments? Do you get better and then worse? Do you easily relapse? If this is the case then you probably then have Mycobacteria which is protecting the Candida and causing it to remain in place.

How to Kill Mycobacteria in the Digestive System

After much trial and error, we have determined that combining Phase 0 of the Candida protocol with several products from WEI Labs and a product best described as an "enzyme disrupter" that can digest the slime that coats the Mycobacteria is the best and most effective treatment plan. This protocol is taken for a minimum time of six months to ensure complete removal. However, the duration of the program can be adjusted based on the home urine test results. Most patients seem to hit the peak of die-off after about two weeks on the treatment plan. It is normal to start feeling the die-off after the first four days of the plan. The four products used in Phase 0 have a flushing and sweeping effect like the products from WEI Labs, and both stop the pathogenic activity of the bacteria while dissolving the slime coating. The "Disrupter" is simply used to digest as much slime as possible in order to complete expose the Myocbacteria to the attach of your 'Killers."

The discovery of and plan to eliminate MYCOBATERIA is the biggest since Candida itself. It answers why some people have not gotten the results we hoped for over the last few years.

Candida Diets

The Candida Diet is a necessary evil, as many of my patients will agree. If you are a Candida sufferer, the diet is something that "you can't live with, yet you can't live without." The diet is feared, hated, despised, misunderstood, and often can make the difference between the success and failure in the elimination of the yeasty beast! The purpose of this article is not to explain what the Candida Diet is. This can actually be found on our website in the "patient only section," or by simply searching the Candida Diet on the internet. The purpose here is to explain why it is important! I will also explain how the diet is generally healthier than most diets that are being followed in the 21st Century.

The Candida Diet is low in carbohydrates, low in sugar, and generally low in fermented foods like vinegar and alcoholic beverages. Candida feeds on sugars. Sugars make it grow and strengthen its adherence to the intestinal lining. While on a Candida Diet, the total amount of carbohydrates for the day should not exceed 150 grams.

At the Biamonte Center, we use three versions of the Candida Diet that range between 30-50 grams, 60-90 grams, and 100-150 grams of total carbohydrates for the day. Avoiding sugar and alcohol are the most important factors. These substances can cause the fastest and greatest increase in Candida growth. They are the most dangerous. Starches come next. Starches convert to sugars in your body. Candida can feed on healthy sugars just the same as it can on junk food. Many of our patients will notice that sweet fruits will flare their symptoms just as noticeably as junk foods! When eating starches (carbohydrates), choosing those foods that have a lower "glycemic index" rating is best.

The glycemic index is a scale that rates how fast a food converts into sugar in the blood stream. Examples of the glycemic index can easily be found on the internet. Fermented foods, like soy sauce and vinegar can be important to avoid, especially if the person has reactionary symptoms from the food. These foods often produce an allergic reaction in the Candida sufferer's intestinal tract which can upset the good flora and the intestinal immune response. Foods from the fungus family like mushrooms can be allergens in the same manner as the fermented foods.

Foods high in yeast can have a similar effect to fermented foods and the foods from the fungal family. Foods that contain yeast do not contain Candida. They contain baker's yeast. This is not Candida. These foods can aggravate Candida by causing allergic reactions, but they cannot cause Candida.

The Candida Diet, though apparently restrictive, is actually higher in nutrients than the diet of the average American. In fact, the Candida Diet is very similar to "The South Beach Diet," "The Zone," and "The Hunter/Gatherer Diet" (also known as the "Paleolithic Diet").

There are races of people who are all slimmer, stronger, and faster than us. They all have straight teeth and perfect eyesight. Arthritis, diabetes, hypertension, heart disease, stroke, depression, schizophrenia, and cancer are absolute rarities to them. These people are the last 84 tribes of hunter-gatherers in the world. They share a secret that is over two million years old. Their secret is their diet: a diet that has changed little from that of the first humans two million years ago and from that of human predecessors up to seven million years ago. Theirs is the diet upon which humanity evolved: the diet that is coded for in our genes. It has some major differences to the diet of "civilization." You are in for a few big surprises.

The diet is usually referred to as the "Paleolithic Diet," referring to a Paleolithic or Stone Age era. It is also referred to as the "Stone Age Diet," "Cave Man Diet," or the "Hunter/Gatherer Diet." More romantic souls like to think of it as the diet that was eaten in the "Garden of Eden," and they are correct in thinking so. For millions of years, humans and their relatives have eaten meat, fish, fowl, and the leaves, roots, and fruits of many plants. One big obstacle to getting more calories from the environment is the fact that many plants are inedible. Grains, beans, and potatoes are full of energy, but are all inedible in the raw state as they contain many toxins. There is no doubt about that. Please don't try to eat them raw. They can make you very sick.

Around 10,000 years ago, an enormous breakthrough was made, a breakthrough that was to change the course of history, and our diet, forever. This breakthrough was the discovery that cooking these foods made them edible. The heat destroyed enough toxins to render them edible. Grains include wheat, corn, barley, rice, sorghum, millet, and oats. Grain based foods also include products such as flour, bread, noodles, and pasta. The cooking of grains, beans, and potatoes had an enormous effect on our food intake, perhaps doubling the number of calories that humans could obtain from the plant foods in their environment.

Grains, beans, and potatoes (GBP) share the following important characteristics:

- They are all toxic when raw. There is no doubt about this; it is a fact that no competent source would dispute. Grains, beans, and potatoes can be extremely dangerous, and it is important never to eat them raw or undercooked. Their toxins include enzyme blockers, lectins, and other types. I will talk about them in detail later as they are very important.
- Cooking destroys most but not all of the toxins. Insufficient cooking can lead to sickness such as acute gastroenteritis.
- They are all rich sources of carbohydrate and, once cooked, this is often rapidly digestible, giving it a high glycemic index (sugar

spike).

- They are extremely poor sources of vitamins (particularly vitamins A, B-group, folic acid, and C), minerals, antioxidants, and phytosterols.

Therefore diets high in grains, beans, and potatoes (GBP):

- contain toxins in small amounts
- have a high glycemic index (i.e. have a similar effect to raw sugar on blood glucose levels)
- are low in many vitamins, minerals, antioxidants, and phytosterols (i.e. they are the original "empty calories")
- have problems caused by the GBP displacing other foods

As grains, beans and potatoes form such a large proportion of the modern diet, you can now understand why it is so common for people to feel they need supplements or that they need to detoxify (i.e. that they have toxins in their system). Indeed both feelings are absolutely correct. The essentials of the Paleolithic Diet are:

- Eat none of the following: (Note the following is not the Candida Diet this information is present in order to compare the Candida Diet to the Paleolithic Diet.)
  - grains- including bread, pasta, noodles
  - beans- including string beans, kidney beans, lentils, peanuts, snow-peas, and peas
  - potatoes
  - dairy products
  - sugar
- Eat the following: (Note the following is not the Candida Diet- this information is present in order to compare the Candida Diet to the Paleolithic Diet.)
  - meat, chicken, and fish
  - eggs
  - fruits

- vegetables (especially root vegetables, but definitely not including potatoes or sweet potatoes)
- nuts, e.g. walnuts, Brazil nuts, macadamia, almond- Do not eat peanuts (a bean) or cashews (a family of their own)
- berries- strawberries, blueberries, raspberries, etc.

Try to increase your intake of

- root vegetables- carrots, turnips, parsnips, rutabagas, Swedes
- organ meats: liver and kidneys (I accept that many people find these unpalatable and won't eat them.)

This diet strongly resembles the typical Candida Diet, which in fact is higher in nutrient density than most diets that are followed by the average American. From a layman's point of view, we can say that we use the diet to starve Candida in order to kill it. From a more scientific point of view, sugars, when metabolized by Candida cells, help Candida to adhere to the intestinal lining in order to hold on and keep its grip on you! Therefore, the avoidance of sugars can weaken the grip that the Candida has on your intestinal lining. Sugars also make up and comprise the outer most layers of the yeast cells. A flip to this statement is the sugar, "Mannose." The sugar, Mannose, is currently being researched by this author, as it has shown the ability to block the adherence of Candida to the vaginal lining and perhaps the intestinal lining.

Candida above all is a yeast/fungus so it can be considered vegetation, like a mushroom. Like brewer's yeast, it metabolizes sugars and converts them to toxic alcohols called aldehydes. Many of the symptoms of Candida are produced by this toxic alcohol, the toxic proteins called antigens, mycotoxins (fungal toxins), and the neurological toxins (neurotoxins) that the Candida produces. When Candida is fed sugars, it not only strengthens its grip on you, but it also produces more of these toxins. Starches and carbohydrates are naturally broken down and converted to sugars by your own body. This is normal for your health.

However, Candida will eat these sugars as well. Fermented foods contain predigested sugars and substances that react like allergens with your Candida. So sugars, starches, alcohol, and fermented foods feed Candida and make it worse! They also make it harder for medicines to kill Candida.

Diet, however, rarely causes Candida. Candida is usually caused by antibiotics, steroids, birth control pills, and other drugs. However, a diet high in sugar, starch, and alcohol, consumed during a period of extreme stress can bring Candida about as if one took these medications.

At the Biamonte Center, the Candida Diet is used to weaken the Candida by starving it. This makes the Candida more susceptible to the anti-yeast/ anti- fungal substances that we use. The Candida Diet is not used to kill the Candida as its own weapon. Diet very rarely can eliminate Candida. Candida grows a root system into your blood vessels. Here it taps into you blood and feeds on blood glucose and other nutrients. There is always enough blood glucose to keep the Candida alive despite the patient being on a low carbohydrate diet or even if you fasted. Fasting cannot kill Candida! This is because even when you fast, your body must keep a normal level of glucose (blood sugar) circulating for your brain and muscles to work. However, the low carb diet weakens it, like a weed which has had little water for some time. Even when it is barely alive, Candida can continue to survive. And if "watered and fed properly," could grow again, returning to its former glory.

This is a very important concept to understand when we consider the importance and place the diet treatment holds in the elimination of Candida.

DIET RARELY ELIMINATES CANDIDA. ITS PURPOSE IS TO MAKE THE CANDIDA WEAKER SO THAT THE MEDICINES CAN TOTALLY DESTROY IT!

When you cheat on the diet, the Candida can temporarily increase. If you cheat for one day on the diet but continue the Candida rotation and Phase 0, little will happen to set you back. Any increase in growth can be reduced within one to two days. The more you cheat, the more Candida grows. If you do the program but do not follow the diet, either no progress will be made, or you will continually feel ill from feeding the Candida, then making it grow, and then killing it and becoming toxic from the dead Candida wastes!

So when you cheat a day or so here and there on the diet, it does not defeat the entire program, providing that you stay on the anti-fungal rotation and Phase 0.

Why are Gluten and Milk Excluded in the Candida Diets?

Many of the Candida diets also suggest excluding Gluten and Casein (milk protein) from the diet. What isn't explained is why. It is observed that most, but not all, Candida patients worsen when eating these foods.

A possible theory as to why, is that an underlying allergy to these foods causes damage to the intestinal condition and damage to the intestinal villi occurs. These villi are finger- like hairs that absorb nutrients that pass through the intestines. This damage causes putrefaction and decay of food in the intestines due to malabsorption.

In that case, the Candida is provided with food, so it can continue to proliferate. This can also suppress normal, healthy flora and the intestinal immune response. The underlying problem is gluten-induced intestinal damage, but because the Candida is easier to identify, the underlying pathology is missed. Candida could easily eat these foods and release allergens as a by-product of its metabolism, which causes intestinal allergies and further degrades the intestinal flora.

Weight Gain and Candida

"It's Not Your Fault"

If you have failed to lose weight despite following a diet exactly, it could be due to Candida. The late Dr. Robert Atkins, an international expert on the low carbohydrate diet, says in his books that Candida or low thyroid function can prevent weight loss despite a low carbohydrate diet. Candida adversely affects your metabolism and interferes with many hormones, nutrients, and the body's ability to burn fat!

One of the major secondary problems associated with Candida Albicans is weight gain. A number of the problems associated with losing weight and staying with a diet are due to Candida Albicans. A person with Candida Albicans will often crave sugar and simple carbohydrates because this is the main source of nutrients for yeast. Mood swings and depression are often associated with the rapid change in blood sugar levels caused by the yeast. Lower thyroid function, lower Dhea levels, estrogen dominance, and elevated cortisol levels are all typical in someone with chronic Candida. Each of these situations has been known to contribute to weight gain or difficulty losing weight. Focusing on removing Candida Albicans from the body rewards the dieter with a feeling of well-being and weight loss that is steady, sustainable, and healthy. Very often a person trying to lose weight will not be able to do so because of a Candida infection.

A New Miracle Food to Stop Sugar and Carbohydrate Cravings so You Can Stay on The Diet!

Hemp Hearts (Shelled Hemp Seed) is a natural food that is concentrated with all of the required proteins, essential fats, and many vitamins and enzymes, and contains only insignificant quantities of saturated fats and carbohydrates. Because Hemp Hearts provides an excellent balance of proteins and essential fats, people will have less difficulty avoiding the sugar and starchy carbohydrates that cause obesity and many other late onset health problems. Individuals who use Hemp Hearts by eating them in the morning for their nutritional essentials, to increase their energy and reduce their dependence on sugar and carbohydrates and having all day to burn off the calories will always experience profound health benefits.

With the exception of people with diabetes and other conditions which may require individuals to eat more frequently, most people should eat at least four, but usually five, measured tablespoons of Hemp Hearts early each morning, preferably on fruit and yogurt (vegetables for diabetics), but also sometimes on cereal. People who do this frequently report that they are not yet hungry at lunch time and often only slightly hungry at three or four o'clock in the afternoon. Those who are overweight can quite easily limit themselves to a large salad in the afternoon. Because people who eat Hemp Hearts in quantity every morning are nutritionally satisfied, they have less difficulty avoiding foods made with sugar, flour, potatoes, pasta, and rice, and they are less inclined to regain lost weight.

The New Low Carb Boom!

Since the popularity of the "Atkins Diet," many companies have emerged that produce low carb versions of popular snack foods and baked goods. These companies are easily accessed on the internet. In most cases, these foods are perfect for the Candida diet.

Basic Info on Candida Diet

The most common questions we get at the Center are about diet. In a nation riddled with obesity, diabetes, and cardiovascular disease it is not surprising that people are confused about what to eat. What is a healthy diet? Is it low fat? Low carb? Vegetarian? Vegan? Gluten free? Lactose free? Raw?

It seems everywhere you turn you have another expert telling you that their diet is the only way to eat. That's before you even begin to bring an illness like Candida, Leaky Gut, or Autism into the picture. The truth of the matter is that there is no one perfect diet for everyone. If this seems like a strange concept, consider this: You are not the same as your friends, your neighbor, or even your family. Your body has its own particular set of genetics and circumstances that make it unique. What works for one person will not necessarily work for another. Today we will talk about the general building blocks of a healthy diet, there will be a follow up to this article that talks about the specifics of a Candida-safe diet, but you should have this information first.

Hydration: Other than air, this is our body's most basic necessity. A person can actually survive weeks without food, but only days without water. Make sure you drink six to eight glasses of water a day. Notice I said water, not liquids! While it's true you can function with coffee, juice, tea, or soda, your body has to work to distill these to down to what it really wants; useable H_2O. Better to think of other liquids as a treat and to make sure that you get enough pure water (lemon or lime can be added for flavor and electrolytes). I can't tell you how many people have solved low energy, headaches, or die off from our program just by ensuring they got enough water throughout the day.

Protein: Protein is a nutrient needed for growth and maintenance of cells. After water, protein is the most abundant substance in the body. Without protein, our bodies cannot grow, cannot heal and cannot function. Eating protein also supplies certain amino acids (the building blocks of protein) that the human body cannot make itself. For the most part, proteins are found in meats or animal products such as milk or eggs. But it is also available in certain nuts, seeds, and legumes, although in lower concentrations.

Lipids: Lipids are not the same thing as fats. The group of lipids includes fat soluble vitamins like A, D, E, and K. Essential fatty acids, Triglycerides, and Cholesterol. Lipids are probably the most misunderstood portion of nutrition. I could write an entire article on lipids alone, and there are many books on the subject. But for the sake of what's needed in a generally healthy diet, here's what you need to know: Our bodies need fat. One of the most important ways that the body uses lipids is in the makeup of cells. Healthy fats can be found in nuts, seeds, olive oil, avocado, fish oil, and grass fed beef. Lipids play a key role in energy production. When you eat, your body converts any calories it doesn't need to use right away into triglycerides. They are then the body's go-to source of energy between meals. The body can obtain energy from many sources, but Triglycerides store the most energy in the least amount of space. I am sure you're thinking, "Wait a minute, aren't triglycerides bad? I have to keep an eye on them or I'll have a heart attack." We'll get back to them. Keep reading.

Trans fats are one of the few things I will tell people to avoid completely. They are found in most processed foods such as fast food, crackers, packaged cookies, cakes, and the like. Trans fats can be made from many different oils and are usually listed on ingredients as "partially hydrogenated xxx oil." *Partial hydrogenation* is an industrial process used to make perfectly good oil, such as soybean oil, into perfectly bad oil. The process is used to make an oil more solid in order to provide longer shelf-life in baked products, to offer longer fry-life for cooking oils, and to produce a certain kind of texture or "mouthfeel to a product."

If the label says *zero tran-fats* it isn't always true! If the list of ingredients contains includes the words "partially hydrogenated" or "shortening," the product DOES contain trans fat. The FDA allows .5 grams of trans fats or less to be listed as "no trans fats." Trans fats will increase your bad cholesterol, lower your good cholesterol, and harden your arteries. If you avoid these fats and follow the rest of the diet advice below, it is very unlikely you will have the heart and cholesterol problems so many others can't seem to get a handle on.

Nutrient rich roughage: This category of foods is the easiest to explain. It's likely you grew up hearing "eat your vegetables" at every meal. It was great advice. The technical reason that it is very important to consume a good amount of roughage, is that roughage helps keep your digestive system moving by adding fiber and bulk, and thus keeps your body detoxified. A slow moving bowel will leech all your energy and is a haven for parasites and other opportunistic organisms. Greens also contain many antioxidants and are a great source of vitamins and trace minerals. Many people seem to have the idea that these vegetables are "boring" or that eating them is a chore. I personally find vegetables to be my favorite food group. Try new vegetables, like kale, mustard greens, bok choy, and swiss chard. Eat broccoli rabe with olive oil, lemon, and hot pepper or try escarole soup with garlic and white beans, and then tell me that vegetables are boring! I'll bet you won't. Challenge yourself to have a serving of green vegetables at every meal for a week (even breakfast). You will feel full longer, have more energy, and have less craving for processed foods.

Carbohydrates: Strictly speaking, the body does not require many carbohydrates at all. That's not to say carbs don't have their uses or that everyone should be on a no carb diet. Many foods that are rich in vitamins and minerals have a carbohydrate component to them. Carbohydrates are broken down very quickly into glucose. Glucose is your cells' primary source of energy, but they are not the only source (see, triglycerides in lipids section). The more active you are at any given moment, the more energy your body needs to keep functioning while it does the work of running your organs and breaking down lipids and proteins. The problem arises when a person consumes more energy than they need at the time, on a consistent basis.

If you eat a serving of carbohydrates, especially when they are processed, which makes them breakdown faster, your blood glucose levels shoot up almost instantly. In order to maintain the proper levels of sugar in your blood and to prevent the catastrophe of glucose shock, your body releases a hormone called insulin. Insulin is a "master" hormone. If your metabolism were a ship, Insulin would be the captain. When it is released it is a signal for cells in the liver, muscles, and fat tissues to stop doing what they normally would be doing in order to focus on taking in glucose from the blood and storing it as glycogen. (Stop cleaning the deck, stop repairing the sails, grab a bucket and start bailing water!) Glycogen is similar to triglycerides in that it is a molecule that stores energy. The main difference is that it is far less efficient. Now here's the kicker. When Insulin is released, it stops the use of fat as energy; presumably this is because it is better for your body to use the less efficient glycogen first before tapping into its sources of triglycerides which are more valuable to the body since they store more energy in less space. What begins to happen when this occurs regularly is your body gets a massive stockpile of glycogen, which the insulin forces it to use first.

Then those triglycerides start to stockpile too, since you're not just eating carbs, you're eating fats, and now those fat stores start to become more visible on your body, your jeans don't fit well, your energy starts to sag because your body is forced to use lower quality fuel, and you want to move around less. Through all of this, it's likely that you're still eating the same amount of carbohydrates and continuing the vicious cycle.

What can happen next? Insulin resistance. The receptors in your muscles, liver, and fat tissues have had enough of this game. They aren't as quick to jump when the captain says grab the bucket. It takes longer and longer to get the job done, and your body is subject to high glucose levels for too long which will eventually begin to cause problems. If everything isn't brought under control quickly, the ship will sink or a mutiny will occur. Your metabolism can't do its job properly, and you may become diabetic. So what does all this mean to the average person? Should I, or should I not cut carbs? Well the answer is yes and no.

You really should cut out processed carbohydrates (that means white flour, pasta, white rice, white sugar, etc) as they have no nutritional value beyond raising your blood glucose level. No one needs these types of foods, and studies have shown that eating them can cause you to crave them more. However, if you are otherwise healthy, you could eat them in limited amounts. As for other carbohydrates, you should eat them in the form of legumes, whole grains, fruits, and other carbohydrate- and nutrient-rich vegetables such as carrots, cauliflower, and sweet potatoes all in relation to how active you are. An athlete or extremely active individual who is moving around all day, needs to eat a fairly large amount of carbohydrates to keep their energy up. Chances are this type of person does not have huge stock piles of glycogen and triglycerides because they are always moving, and their body is using that energy. Conversely, a person who wakes up, drives to work, sits at work, drives home, is not physically active there, and doesn't exercise needs almost no carbohydrates. It is likely you fall somewhere in the middle. For an active person, having carbs as about 30 percent of your diet is probably sufficient, Just make sure the sources of those carbohydrates are not refined. If you start losing more weight than you should, that's a good indicator that you need to eat more carbohydrates.

1. Concomitant Foods

Concomitant foods are food that produce a reaction only in the presence of an inhalant allergen, usually pollen. The same reaction can also happen in the presence of dust and mold allergens. The following list is used for reference. Please be advised that these foods have the potential of complicating your symptoms. Only you can determine if they bother you. If you notice that these foods provoke your symptoms or make them worse, avoid them. If you are free of symptoms, enjoy these foods.

<u>Tree season begins mid-February and ends in June</u>

Elm - Milk

Oak – Egg, Lettuce, Apple, Mint, Chestnut, Chocolate, Pears

<u>Grass season begins in May and ends in July</u>

General Grasses: Timothy (specific), Wheat, Apple, Legumes (peas, beans, grains, soybeans), Carrots, Corn, Celery, Pears, Cottonseed (cooking fats)

<u>Ragweed season begins August and ends with the first good frost</u>

[Completely avoid the following]: Milk, Melons (honey dew, cantaloupe), Mint, Cucumber, Zucchini, Chamomile

[Eat with caution]: Banana, Sunflower seeds, Pumpkin, Echinacea, Potentially any vine fruit or vegetable

<u>Dust happens all year Mold is in the environment all year</u>

Peanuts, Mushrooms, Peanut butter, Aged cheeses (esp. blue cheese), Shrimp, Coffee, Oysters, Fermented beverages, Snails, Black Tea (use green tea instead)

2. Eat any sugar alcohol lately?

If you've looked lately at the “Nutrition Facts” panel on a pack of sugar-free gum or candy, you might be surprised to see that it contains “sugar alcohol.” Don't let the name fool you. These ingredients were given this consumer-friendly name because part of their structure resembles sugar and part is similar to alcohol. Sugar alcohols do not contain ethanol, which is found in alcoholic beverages.

What is sugar alcohol?

Sugar alcohols, also known as polyols, are ingredients used as bulking agents and sweeteners. They occur naturally in foods and come from plant products such as fruits and berries. As a sugar substitute, they provide fewer calories (about a half to one-third less calories) than regular sugar. This is because they are converted to glucose more slowly, require little or no insulin to be metabolized, and don't cause sudden increases in blood sugar. This makes them popular among individuals with diabetes; however, their use is becoming more common by just about everyone. You may be consuming them and not even know it.

Identifying Sugar Alcohols

Common sugar alcohols are mannitol, sorbitol, xylitol, lactitol, isomalt, maltitol, and hydrogenated starch hydrolysates (HSH). Sugar alcohols are not commonly used in home food preparation but are found in many processed foods. Food products labeled "sugar-free," including hard candies, cookies, chewing gums, soft drinks, and throat lozenges often consist of sugar alcohols. They are frequently used in toothpaste and mouthwash, too.

Check carbohydrates

So why are sugar alcohols used so often? For one thing, they help to provide a sweet flavor to food in many products marketed towards individuals with diabetes. But, beware! There is often the misconception that all sugar alcohol-containing products are "free foods." Some of these products may still contain significant amounts of carbohydrates. It's important to check the food label for the total carbohydrate contained in the product and to talk with a registered dietitian to determine how it will best fit into your meal plan.

If a manufacturer uses the term "sugar free" or "no added sugar," they must list the grams of sugar alcohols. If more than one sugar alcohol is used in a product, the "Nutrition Facts" panel will list the amount of sugar alcohol it contains under the total carbohydrate. If just one sugar alcohol is used, the label will list its specific name, for example, "mannitol" or "hydrogenated starch hydrolysates."

Pros and cons of sugar alcohols

On the *positive* side, sugar alcohols contain fewer calories (1.5 - 3 calories per gram) than sugar (4 calories per gram), and they do not cause tooth decay like sugar does. Therefore, many "sugar-free" gums including Trident® and Extra® are made with sugar alcohols. Sugar alcohols also add texture to foods, retain moisture better, and prevent foods from browning when they are heated.

Unfortunately, there are some *negatives* associated with sugar alcohols. The most common side effect is the possibility of bloating and diarrhea when sugar alcohols are eaten in excessive amounts. There is also some evidence that sugar alcohols, much like fructose (natural fruit sugar) in fruit and fruit juice, can cause a "laxative effect." Weight gain has been seen when these products are overeaten. The American Diabetes Association claims that sugar alcohols are acceptable in a moderate amount but should not be eaten in excess. Some people with diabetes, especially Type I diabetics, have found that their blood sugars rise if sugar alcohols are eaten in uncontrolled amounts.

Sugar Alcohols vs. Artificial Sweeteners

Sugar alcohols and artificial sweeteners, such as saccharin (Sweet & Low®) and aspartame (Equal® or NutraSweet®) are not one and the same. One difference between the two types of sugar substitutes is that the artificial sweeteners contain zero calories whereas sugar alcohols contain about 2.6 calories per gram. Another issue is diabetes management. Artificial sweeteners do not contain carbohydrates, so they do not cause blood sugar to elevate, whereas sugar alcohols have some effect on blood sugar. Overall, both can be useful in diabetes management when used properly.

Forms of sugar alcohol:

Mannitol occurs naturally in pineapples, olives, asparagus, sweet potatoes, and carrots. It is extracted from seaweed for use in food manufacturing. Mannitol has 50 - 70 percent of the relative sweetness of sugar which means more must be used to equal the sweetness of sugar. Mannitol lingers in the intestines for a long time and therefore often causes bloating and diarrhea.

Sorbitol is found naturally in fruits and vegetables. It is manufactured from corn syrup. Sorbitol has only 50 percent of the relative sweetness of sugar which means twice as much must be used to deliver a similar amount of sweetness to a product. It has less of a tendency to cause diarrhea compared to mannitol. It is often an ingredient in sugar-free gums and candies.

Xylitol is also called "wood sugar" and occurs naturally in straw, corncobs, fruit, vegetables, cereals, mushrooms, and some cereals. Xylitol has the same relative sweetness as sugar. It is found in chewing gums.

Lactitol has about 30 - 40 percent of sugar's sweetening power, but its taste and solubility profile resembles sugar, so it is often found in sugar-free ice cream, chocolate, hard and soft candies, baked goods, sugar-reduced preserves, and chewing gums.

Isomalt is 45 - 65 percent as sweet as sugar and does not tend to lose its sweetness or break down during the heating process. Isomalt absorbs little water, so it is often used in hard candies, toffee, cough drops, and lollipops.

Maltitol is 75 percent as sweet as sugar. It is used in sugar-free hard candies, chewing gum, chocolate-flavored desserts, baked goods, and ice cream because it gives a creamy texture to foods.

Hydrogenated starch hydrolysates (HSH) are produced by the partial hydrolysis of corn. HSH are nutritive sweeteners that provide 40 - 90 percent of the sweetness of sugar. HSH do not crystallize and are used extensively in confections, baked goods, and mouthwashes.

3. Prohibited foods

Gluten grains (wheat, oats barley), dairy except butter, sugar in all forms (including agave, honey, beet sugar, maple syrup etc.), alcohol, vinegar (except apple cider vinegar), soda, peanuts, all fruits not listed, coffee, caffeinated teas. Fermented foods, yogurt, many condiments, soy sauce, miso soup, brewer's yeast.

4. Substitutions

Sugar substitutions:

A common question is what sugar substitutions can be used while on the diet. The following are generally safe, but be aware that, like anything, that they should still be used in moderation. Xylitol, Stevia, Splenda (liquid, powdered forms usually contain glucose), Glycerin.

Substitutions for flour and bread crumbs: (use sparingly)

Ground nuts, seeds to make a meal, sesame seeds, shredded coconut, dry minced onion, potato flour, corn flour, buckwheat flour, brown rice flour, whole-grain millet flour, whole-grain amaranth flour.

THE BIAMONTE CENTER BASIC CANDIDA DIET

This diet can include up to 120 grams of carbohydrate. It is for the average case of Candida. (On the urine test an Oxidata 3 or less, with a Dysbiosis marker of floating to heavy curdled will match this diet)

VEGETABLES (must be washed using a fruit/vegetable disinfectant product as available in the health food store to avoid mold, bacteria reactions, and parasite reinfestation.)

(UNLIMITED EACH DAY)

Beet Greens, Dandelion Greens, Boston Lettuce, Romaine Lettuce, Iceberg Lettuce, Chicory, Arugula, Watercress, Kale, Escarole, Swiss Chard, Collards, Spinach, Celery, Cauliflower, Broccoli, all Cabbages, Bok Choy, Fennel, Asparagus, all Sprouts, Cucumber, Radish, Eggplant, Green Beans, Turnips, Artichokes, Endive, Radicchio, Rhubarb, Zucchini, Garlic, Canned Tomato, all Peppers, Broccoli Rabe.

VEGETABLES IN LIMITED QUANTY (must be washed using a fruit/vegetable disinfectant product as available in the health food store to avoid mold, bacteria reactions and parasite reinfestation)

(2 servings from this group per day)
Scallions ¼ cup per serving, Shallots ¼ cup per serving, Leeks ¼ cup per serving, Onions ¼ cup per serving, Carrots ½ per serving, Tomatoes 1 medium per serving,

(¼ to ½ cup daily)
Chick Peas, Kidney Beans, Lentils, Soy Beans and Black Eyed Peas

(1 serving 2- 3 times per week)
Yam 1 medium, Summer Squash ½ cup, Acorn Squash ½ cup, Spaghetti Squash ½ cup, Peas ½ cup

If you notice any reaction to these foods then remove from diet.

GRAINS
(1/3 cup per day)
Wild Rice, Brown Rice, Millet, Buckwheat, Amaranth

(3/4 cup per day)
Quinoa

(Other)
Mary's Gone Crackers – 6 per day, Arrowhead Mills Puffed Rice, Millet or Kamut - ¼ to ½ cups per day, Bob's Redeye Almond Meal & Tapioca - I serving per day, Arrowhead Mills Organic Buckwheat Flour - 1 serving per day, Orgran All Purpose Rice Crumbs – 1 serving per day

All grains to be used in limited quantities. If you notice any reactions, remove from diet.

NUTS/SEEDS (dry roasted or raw)
(¼- ½ cup per day)
Almonds, Pistachios, Hazel Nuts, Brazil Nuts, Macadamia Nuts, Pecans,

Walnuts, Pumpkin Seeds, Sesame Seeds, Hemp Seeds, Butters made from the nuts/seeds listed.

Should be removed from diet if any of these foods cause constipation.

OILS (unlimited)
Extra Virgin Olive Oil, Virgin Coconut Oil, Macadamia Nut Oil, Walnut Oil

DAIRY
Unsalted Butter *UNSALTED BUTTER
Heavy Cream – ¼ cup daily, Goat or sheep cheeses ,Ricotta Cheese – ¼ cup daily

(All dairy to be used in limited quantities. If you notice any reactions, remove from diet. Not to be used if lactose intolerant)

MEATS (unlimited)(must be well cooked to avoid reinfestation)
Organic Grass Fed, Hormone & Antibiotic Free preferred
Beef, Bacon (Nitrite Free / Wood Smoked), Sausage (Nitrite Free), Lamb, Pork, Veal, All Wild Game

POULTRY (unlimited)(must be well cooked to avoid bacterial infection and parasitic reinfestation) Organic Grass Fed, Hormone & Antibiotic Free preferred
Chicken, Turkey, Cornish Game Hen, Duck, All Wild Poultry, Eggs

FISH (unlimited)(Must be well cooked to avoid parasite reinfestation)
Wild Caught Only (Avoid Tuna, Swordfish and other large fish)

FRUITS (must be washed using a fruit/vegetable disinfectant product as available in the health food store to avoid mold, bacteria reactions and parasite reinfestation)

(2 servings per day)
STRAWBERRIES ½- 1 cup, Black & Blueberries ½- 1 cup, Raspberries ½- 1

cup, Boysenberries ½- 1 cup, Cherries ½- 1 cup, Granny Smith Apples - 1 per day; Lemons, Limes, Grapefruit ½ per day.

EXTRACTS

Almond, Lemon, Orange and Vanilla

SWEETNERS

(Limit to 3 servings per day. Serving size indicated on product label)
Xylitol, Truvia, Stevia

(Remove from the diet should you notice any reaction to them.)

BEVERAGES

Consuming adequate amounts of water is an essential part of the program. Recommended amount is half your weight in ounces. For example, if you weigh 180 pounds, you must consume 90 ounces of water daily.

Other beverages include:

Herbal Teas, Coffee, English Teas, Green Tea, Club Soda, Sparkling Water, Flavored Seltzer, Diluted Unsweetened Cranberry Juice, Coconut Water, Unsweetened *Almond Breeze* Almond Milk, Unsweetened *Blue Diamond* Coconut Milk

OTHER/MISCELLANEOUS

Unsweetened Cocoa Powder, Sea Salt, Pepper (All Types), All Herbs (Dry & Fresh), Coleman's Powdered Dry Mustard, Olives in Oil or Water, Capers in Oil or Water, Horseradish (Fresh Grated Raw), Taj Ethnic Gourmet Indian Sauces, Organic Dark Chocolate (70% Cocoa or Higher. Only 4 ounces per day)

MUST AVOIDS

1. **Alcohol**
2. **Sugar Sweetened Sodas**

3. **Sugar in all forms** including white cane sugar, Honey, Molasses, Barley Malt, Date Sugar, Manitol, Maltose, High Fructose Corn Sugar. Note very small amounts of some sweeteners may be acceptable in certain recipes as the amounts ingested per serving will be very small. However these sugars are never to be used as any prominent or significant portion of your diet. If they are used it should be in only "tiny amounts." Overuse of any sweet substance can result in relapse or prolonged use of the diet.
4. **Yeast Product**, such as Breads, Cakes, Cookies, Muffins, Etc. Yeast containing products don't feed Candida but are likely sources of allergens that stress the immune system and can further imbalance the GI tract.
5. **Dairy; Milk, Cheese**, (except for those previously listed), **Ice Cream**.
6. **Grains;** Wheat, Oats, Barley and Rye all contain Gluten or Gluten-like substances. Gluten is highly allergic to Candida patients. CORN may contain too much sugar for a Candida patient and should be avoided.
7. **Fermented Foods**; Yogurt, vinegar, mustard, horse radish, miso, soy sauce, brewer's yeast, commercial mayonnaise, pickled foods etc.
8. **Mushrooms and any edible fungus.**
9. **Dried Fruits.**
10. **Cashews**; Can be constipating.
11. **Peanuts;** Contain Aflatoxin B which is highly toxic to Candida patients.

THE BIAMONTE CENTER ADVANCED CANDIDA DIET

This diet can include up to 80 grams of carbohydrate, it is for the average case of Candida. Select and balance meals from foods listed herein. Eat at least three meals a day or six small ones, if preferred. Snacks are permitted only from among foods listed herein. Balance protein intake with green leafy vegetables in at least one generous green salad daily.

BREAD / CEREALS: None of any kind.

DAIRY PRODUCTS: Butter and eggs-unlimited.

FISH: (Must be cooked well to avoid parasite infestation) (Fresh fish only) (May be broiled or fried, baked or broiled. Do not use bread crumbs or flour) Cod, Flounder, Haddock, Halibut, Herring, Mackerel, Perch, Salmon, Sardines, Trout, Snapper, Shell fish, Squid & Octopus.

MEATS: (Must be cooked well to avoid parasite infestation) (Bake, broil, grill or sauté. Organic Organ meats also allowed) Beef, Lamb, Veal, Pork & Poultry.

VEGETABLES (Unlimited)(must be washed using a fruit/vegetable disinfectant product as available in the health food store to avoid mold, bacteria reactions and parasite reinfestation). Artichokes, Asparagus, Green beans, Broccoli rabe, Beet greens, Broccoli, Cabbage, Cauliflower, Celery, Swiss Chard, Chicory, Chives, Collards, Cucumbers, Dandelion, Eggplant, Endive, Escarole, Fennel, Watercress, All Herbs, Kale, All lettuces, Mustard greens, Okra, Green peppers, Radishes, Rhubarb, Spinach, Squash (summer), Tomatoes fresh or canned, Turnip greens, Watercress, Zucchini, Olives (in oil or water) & Capers (in oil or water).

FRUITS: (must be washed using a fruit/vegetable disinfectant product as available in the health food store to avoid mold, bacteria reactions and parasite reinfestation). Granny Smith apples, Blueberries, Strawberries, Raspberries, Avocado, Lemons and limes

MISCELLANEOUS:

Salad dressings made from lime, lemon juice, and olive oil, organic stocks such as beef, chicken or onion, olives (ripe or green), mustard (dry only), hard-boiled eggs, fresh nuts-walnuts, pecans and almonds, stevia may be used, seeds pumpkin and sesame.

BEVERAGES:
Herb teas-unsweetened, Coffee and tea in moderation.

AVOID ALL FOODS CONTAINING ADDED SUGAR OR STARCH:

- No cereals, cereal products, bread stuffs, cakes, cookies, pies, candy, ice cream, etc. No mayonnaise, cider vinegar and no cashews.
- No milk, tomato juice, V-8 juice. No colas of any kind.
- No canned, condensed, evaporated or sweetened milk. No alcohol in any form. No sugar free soft drinks.
- No canned, sweetened, or dried fruits of any kind.
- *Avoid Tuna and Swordfish. Note ones mercury levels can determine whether these fish are desirable.

<u>THE BIAMONTE CENTER CAVEMAN CANDIDA DIET</u>

This diet can include up to 40 to 60 grams of carbohydrate, it is for the average case of Candida. (On the urine test a positive Indican of 2 or higher, Oxidata 4 or higher, with a Dysbiosis marker of heavy curdled will match this diet)

Select and balance meals from foods listed herein. Eat at least three meals a day or six small ones, if preferred. Snacks are permitted only from among foods listed herein. Balance protein intake with green leafy vegetables in at least one generous green salad daily.

BREAD / CEREALS: None of any kind.

DAIRY PRODUCTS: Butter and eggs-unlimited.

FISH: (Fresh and must be well cooked to avoid parasite reinfestation) Cod, Flounder, Haddock, Halibut, Herring, Mackerel, Perch, Salmon,

Sardines, Trout, Snapper, Shell fish, Squid & Octopus (May be broiled or fried, baked or broiled. Do not use bread crumbs or flour.)

MEATS: (must be well cooked to avoid parasite reinfestation) Beef, Lamb, Veal, Pork, Poultry all (Bake, broil, grill or sauté. Organic Organ meats also allowed.)

VEGETABLES: unlimited (must be washed using a fruit/vegetable disinfectant product as available in the health food store to avoid mold, bacteria reactions and parasite reinfestation) Artichokes. Asparagus, Green beans, Broccoli rabe, Beet greens, Broccoli, Cabbage, Cauliflower, Celery, Swiss Chard, Chicory, Chives. Collards, Cucumbers, Dandelion, Eggplant, Endive, Escarole, Fennel, Watercress, All Herbs, Kale, ALL lettuces, Mustard greens, Okra, Green peppers, Radishes, Rhubarb, Spinach, Squash (summer), Tomatoes fresh or canned, Turnip greens, Watercress, Zucchini, Olives in oil or water, Capers in oil or water.

MISCELLANEOUS: Salad dressings made from lime, lemon juice, and olive oil, Organic stocks such as beef, chicken or onion, Olives (ripe or green), Mustard (dry only), Hard-boiled eggs, Fresh nuts-walnuts, pecans and almonds, Stevia , Seeds pumpkin and sesame.

BEVERAGES:
Herb teas-unsweetened. Coffee and tea in moderation.

AVOID ALL FOODS MADE WITH OR CONTAINING SUGAR OR STARCH: No cereals, cereal products, bread stuffs, cakes, cookies, pies, candy, ice cream, etc. No mayonnaise, cider vinegar and no cashews. No milk, tomato juice, V-8 juice. No colas of any kind. No canned, condensed, evaporated or sweetened milk. No alcohol in any form. No sugar free soft drinks. No canned, sweetened, or dried fruits of any kind.

*Avoid Tuna and Swordfish. Note ones mercury levels can determine whether these fish are desirable.

DIET FOR "LEAKY GUT"

When intestinal permeability is present, the intestinal tract can become very allergic, inflamed, and sensitive. Sometimes fiber, which is normally a healthy part of the diet, may create further irritation and produce excess fermentation or gas. The leaky gut diet is similar to the standard Candida Diet with the exception that refined sugars, alcohol, and fermented foods must be more strictly avoided.

A temporary reduction in the following foods would be necessary:

- Raw vegetables
- Raw fruits
- Bran
- Whole grain cereals
- Fiber supplements if they are found to irritate.
- Fermented foods such as vinegar, olives, pickles, yogurt, kefir etc.
- All alcoholic beverages.
- All refined sugars
- Fish pastes
- Sauerkraut
- Sherry Vinegar
- Sour Milk
- Sour Cream
- Soy Sauce
- Breads
- Cheeses
- Kimchi
- Miso
- Tempeh
- Tofu

Cooked vegetables particularly cooked greens are best. Fruits may be steamed or baked.

FLORA DIET (BLOOD TYPE A)

Introduce yogurt, Kiefer, Miso, and other Lactic Acid fermented foods to the diet. Eat at least three servings of these foods a day. (See below for more info on "Lacto Fermented Foods).

1. Increase fruits such as apples, melons, berries, pears, and peaches to at least three servings a day.
2. Increase grain products such as whole grains, sugar free cereals, Non Gluten, and yeast free breads and baked goods to three servings per day. Don't add these foods if your blood type is "O."
3. Eat at least one artichoke per day.
4. Eat two to three servings of beans, peas, or lentils per day.
5. Increase your salads, cooked vegetables, and vegetable-based soups in order to make up at least 65 percent of your diet.
6. Decrease animal protein such as red meat, poultry, fish, and eggs to two servings per day.
7. Decrease animal fats such as butter, lard, cream, bacon, and fatty meats to five servings per week.

More info on Lacto Fermented Foods

A partial list of lacto-fermented vegetables from around the world is sufficient to prove the universality of this practice. In Europe the principle lacto-fermented food is sauerkraut. Described in Roman texts, it was prized for both for its delicious taste as well as its medicinal properties. Cucumbers, beets, and turnips are also traditional foods for lacto-fermentation. Less well known are ancient recipes for pickled herbs, sorrel leaves, and grape leaves. In Russia and Poland one finds pickled green tomatoes, peppers, and lettuces. Lacto-fermented foods form part of Asian cuisines as well. The peoples of Japan, China, and Korea make pickled preparations of cabbage, turnip, eggplant, cucumber, onion, squash, and carrot. Korean kimchi, for example, is a lacto-fermented condiment of cabbage with other vegetables and seasonings that is eaten on a daily basis, and no Japanese meal is complete without a portion of pickled vegetable. American tradition includes many types of relishes -- corn relish, cucumber relish, watermelon rind – all of which were no doubt originally lacto-fermented products. The pickling of fruit is less well known but, nevertheless, is found in many traditional cultures. The Japanese prize pickled umeboshi plums, and the peoples of India traditionally fermented fruit with spices to make chutneys. Lacto-fermented condiments are easy to make. Fruits and vegetables are first washed and cut up, mixed with salt and herbs or spices, and then pounded briefly to release juices. They are then pressed into an air tight container. Salt inhibits putrefying bacteria for several days until enough lactic acid is produced to preserve the vegetables for many months. The amount of salt can be reduced or even eliminated if whey is added to the pickling solution. Rich in lactic acid and lactic-acid-producing bacteria, whey acts as an inoculant, reducing the time needed for sufficient lactic acid to be produced to ensure preservation. Use of whey will result in consistently successful pickling; it is essential for pickling fruits. During the first few days of fermentation, the vegetables are kept at room temperature; afterwards, they must be placed in a cool, dark place for long-term preservation.

How long do have to stay on these diets?

The length of time that one may be on this diet is anywhere between six and 12 months, depending on the persons individual situations. Factors such as the severity of infestation, how closely you follow the diet, how often you cheat, overall health, preexisting illnesses, genetics, life style, stress, and blood type are all factors that will determine the length of the diet.

The Biamonte Candida Cookbook

BREAKFAST

Candida Safe Syrup

Directions:
Melt 1 tbsp Ghee.
Add:
1 tsp of *Maple Flavoring
6 drops of liquid stevia
a sprinkle of ground cinnamon
a pinch of salt.
Mix well and pour over pancakes.

Coconut/Stevia Syrup

Directions:
Melt a little virgin coconut oil and add stevia to taste for a nice syrup. You may also add cinnamon and/or alcohol-free vanilla.

Pancakes

Ingredients for the mix
2 cups almond meal (or 2½ cups almond flour)
½ cup rice bran
½ cup brown rice flour
tsp. flax meal
2½ tsp. aluminum-free baking powder
1½ tsp. salt (kosher or sea salt)
cinnamon and stevia to taste (optional)

Directions:
Mix everything together well and store in an air-tight container.
Makes about 4 cups, each with about 10 net carbs.

To make 2 servings of pancakes:

Ingredients
1 cup mix
1 egg
½ cup water
½ tsp. canola, nut, or sunflower oil

Directions:
Oil a skillet or griddle and set over medium heat.
Mix all ingredients with a whisk and drop the batter by the

tablespoonful onto the griddle or skillet.
Cook until lightly brown on each side.
Stir the batter between batches to prevent it from settling.

Top with a little Chicolin/stevia, additional cinnamon or nutmeg, or whatever you like!

Zucchini Pancakes (By Lauren Insco)

Ingredients (for approximately 8 pancakes)
2 cups finely grated zucchini
1 egg
¼ tsp. Herbamare
¼ tsp. Celtic sea salt
1/8 tsp. fresh ground pepper
Dash paprika
¼ cup quinoa flour
¼ cup almond flour
¼ cup brown rice flour
Dash red pepper flakes

Directions:
Mix batter together well.
Heat about 4 tbsp. olive oil in a frying pan over medium-low heat.
Drop spoonful of batter, about pancake size, into pan.
Flatten lightly with back of spoon to about ½ - ¾ inch thickness (This isn't necessary but will allow the cakes to cook more evenly then if left as dropped.)
Brown on each side.
Remove to paper towel.

Freezes very well. Reheats well. Delicious! Great texture. I think I figured 7 carbs each

NOTE: I have thought about using this as a base for a pizza crust. I would use the zucchini mixture and make a larger round in the pan. Then I would top it with various meat and veggie toppings and possibly a tomato or pesto type sauce with the right ingredients that you can have on the Candida diet

BAKED GOODS

Bread Recipe

Preheat oven to 350° F

Ingredients

3½ cups almond flour
3 eggs
¼ cup melted butter
1 teaspoon baking soda
1 cup yogurt
¼teaspoon salt

Directions:

Mix all ingredients together in food processor.
Pour into a standard loaf pan.
Bake at 350 F (180 C) for about 45 minutes.
You'll have to test to see when it's done.
Let cool completely before removing from pan to prevent bread from collapsing.

NOTE: May be baked on cookie sheet with sides appro. ¾" high. Allow the dough to spread out to fit the sheet completely.

It's thin and bakes quickly. Maybe 15 minutes.

Cut into bread shaped rectangles which can be sliced through to make two pieces if desired.

Karianne's Bread

by Karianne

Preheat oven to 275° F

Ingredients:

14 oz almond butter
2½ oz butternut squash, cooked
¼ cup oil
eggs
1 tsp baking soda
1 tbsp cinnamon

Directions:

Mix all ingredients together in the food processor.
Pour into loaf pan.
Bake at 275°F for 1½ hours.
SO good!!

Flatbread
From
www.thepantrymouse.com
Preheat oven to 350^{oF}

Ingredients:
2 eggs
3 tbsp water
¾ cup brown rice cooked
¾ cup oat flour (I used quinoa or brown rice flour or almond flour)
4½ tbsp amaranth flour

Directions:
Beat egg and stir into water. Add rice and flours.
Add enough boiling water to make batter the consistency of cream). Pour into an oiled 8" pan and spread batter evenly. Bake at 350 F for 25 minutes. Serve warm after cutting into squares.

NOTE: This was excellent! I have used it for sandwiches (used some delicious mustard made with apple cider vinegar and arugula and some organic lunch meat), and I have used it with unsalted butter on top when everyone else around me was having French bread and I couldn't stand it.

I have found many delicious recipes on the www.bodyecologydiet.com website, as well as the www.wholeapproach.com website for Candida sufferers.

Pumpernickel Bread

Gluten Free, Dairy-Free.
Preheat oven to 375°F
Set oven rack on second from bottom position.

Ingredients:

2 eggs plus 2 egg whites (large)
¼ cup vegetable oil (Canola)
¼ cup apple cider vinegar
¼ cup dark molasses
1½ cups warm water (105-115°), divided
2 packages Active Dry Yeast
2 tsp sugar
¼ cup warm unsweetened apple juice (105-115°)
2 cups cornstarch
½ cup tapioca flour
¼ cup glutinous rice flour
1 cup light buckwheat flour
1 cup flaxseed meal
¼ cup cocoa
4 tsp Xanthan gum
1 tsp Salt
2 tsp caraway seeds

Directions:

In medium sized bowl (yeast mixture will expand), place ½ cup of the warm water, yeast, and 2 teaspoons of sugar.
Stir until dissolved.
Allow to sit for 10 minutes.
Mixture will become foamy (if not, the yeast is not active should not be used).

In mixing bowl, combine eggs, egg whites, vegetable oil, remaining 1 cup of warm water.

Mix. Add apple cider vinegar, molasses, and apple juice.

Mix.

Mix together all dry ingredients (cornstarch, flours, flaxseed meal, cocoa, Xanthan gum, salt and caraway seeds)

In a large bowl, add dry ingredients and yeast mixture.

Using electric hand mixer, mix on low speed until combined.

Increase speed to high and mix for 4 minutes.

Place dough in Pyrex round casserole dish (size 2L - if in doubt, should hold 8 cups) which has been sprayed with cooking oil.

Cover loosely with plastic wrap and place in a warm, dry location (free of drafts) for 1 hour to allow dough to rise. (Dough will be slightly above rim of pan).

Place in preheated 375°F oven for 65 minutes. After 20 minutes, place foil over top of bread to avoid over-browning crust.

NOTE: This is a hearty pumpernickel that's great for sandwiches and excellent for parties when served with Dill Dip or Spinach Dip. This pumpernickel bread has a nice hearty crust and a soft spongy center. It holds up well when sliced and used for sandwiches, whether toasted or not. It makes for a great traditional complement to spinach dip for parties too. Check out our dill/spinach dip recipe to accompany this.

Small Loaf Simple Nut Bread

Preheat oven to 300^{OF}

Ingredients:

2½ cups almond flour
¼ teaspoon sea salt
½ teaspoon baking soda
3 eggs
1 tbsp sweetener of a few drops of Stevia (if needed)
½ tsp raw apple cider vinegar

Directions:

Put flour, salt and baking soda in bowl.

In separate bowl, whisk eggs, sweetener, and vinegar. Combine bowls and stir contents.

You may needs to add extra water to achieve a medium thickness pourable batter. Pour into non-stick loaf tin. Bake at 300 degrees for 30 minutes.

Tortillas

Serving Size: 12 tortillas

Ingredients:

¾ cup amaranth
¾ cup flaxseed meal
¾ cup brown rice flour
2 teaspoons Celtic sea salt
2 teaspoons butter

¾ cup of water. (Add only a little at a time till right consistency)

Directions:
In a medium sized bowl stir together the flours and salt.

In a small saucepan over high heat, bring the butter and water to a boil and stir until melted.

Pour the liquid into the flour and blend well with a fork or a pastry blender (add only the water you need!).

You may need more flour to make a soft dough.

On a well-floured surface, kneed for about five minutes, adding more brown rice flour as needed.

Divide the dough into 12 pieces and roll each into a ball.

Roll or pat out the dough until as thin as you can get it.

Heat a large cast iron or other heavy pan over high heat until very hot.

Do not add oil.

Cook the tortillas one at a time until brown on one side, then turn and cook until brown on the second side.

Keep them warm in a tea towel until all are cooked.

NOTE: These were very good. There are about 160 carbs in this entire recipe, but I only needed about half a tortilla (I made less than 12) to be satisfied. I have had these with homemade guacamole, some yummy homemade salsa, or with homemade taco seasoned beef with avocado and olives.

Now that is the low fat healthy option, but for something a bit different, shall we say an anti-Candida-diet-approved treat, try making these tortillas into your own **corn chips**. Cut the tortillas into 8 wedges. Heat oil in your saucepan or skillet, say about 1 inch deep. Heat the oil to medium high heat: it should be able to brown a chip in 60 seconds. Cook the tortilla wedges in batches for 1 to 2 minutes or until golden. Drain on paper towels. When cool they can be stored in air tight container.

Non-Dairy "Cheese"

Ingredients:
½ cup water
3 tbsp gelatin
½ cup boiling water

1 cup raw cashews or unsalted cashews
1 tsp onion powder (or more to taste)
1/8 tsp garlic powder (or more to taste)
2 tbsp lemon juice
¾ tsp salt
½ or less of a large red pepper, chopped finely

Directions:
Put gelatin in the half cup water and let dissolve.
In food processor or blender, mix together the remaining ingredients.
Pour boiling water in the gelatin mixture and stir until there are no lumps.
Add gelatin mixture to the food processor and mix until creamy.
Pour into container the size of a loaf pan only more shallow*.
Cover lightly and let cool.
When cool, slice into long narrow chunks, i.e. into four.
Freeze three and keep one on hand for snacking.

NOTE: Tastes great on a sesame rice cracker (sugar free) which you can find in the Chinese Food section of the grocery store or on a Triscuit (sugar free)

*Tupperware sells a loaf pan with a lid: I use the lid

CONDIMENTS/SAUCES

Chocolate Sauce

Ingredients:
1/8 tsp stevia
1 square unsweetened chocolate
3 tbsp butter or margarine
¾ cup skim milk
1 tbsp cornstarch
½ tsp vanilla

Directions:
In small pot over medium heat, melt chocolate and butter.
Add milk, stevia, and vanilla.
Put cornstarch in a little dish; add some of the milk mixture, blend together until no lumps remain, then pour it back into the pot.
Cook until slightly thickened.
Makes about 1 cup.

Green Sauce

Ingredients:
1 onion
5 cloves garlic
1 tsp of dry coriander

water (enough for proper consistency)
handful fresh coriander and parsley
salt to taste

Directions:
Sautee onion. Add zucchini, garlic, salt, dry coriander, and about 1 cup of water.
Cook until zucchini is soft. Let cool. Add fresh coriander and parsley. Add water until you produce the required consistency.

NOTE: Great with chicken. As I was eating it I was amazed at how much it tasted like avocado, so it would make a great avocado substitute

Mayonnaise

Ingredients:
¾ cup oil
1 egg
2 tablespoons raw unpasteurized apple cider vinegar
1/8 tsp. dry mustard
½ tsp salt
dash pepper
garlic and onion powder (to taste)

Directions:
Add all ingredients except oil to blender.
Begin mixing, slowly drizzling the oil in till gone.
Occasionally stop and scrape down the sides if needed.
Stores well for two weeks in refrigerator.

Lentil Pâté

Ingredients:
1 tbsp olive oil
1 cup chopped onion
cloves minced garlic
1 tsp. sage
1 tsp. thyme
1 1/2 cups cooked and drained lentils
dash of cayenne pepper or to taste

Directions:
Heat the oil in a skillet. Add the onion and garlic, and sauté slowly over low heat for about 15 minutes. Add sage and thyme and continue to sauté for about 5 minutes longer. Place the cooked lentils in a food processor or blender. Add the sautéed vegetables and cayenne pepper to the lentil mixture and puree/blend. Transfer the pate mixture to a bowl and chill about an hour.

NOTE: I've chilled this mixture in mini loaf pans and also in fancier "Tupperware"-type molds.

Pesto

Ingredients:
1/3 cup organic cold pressed olive oil
¼ cup organic parsley
½ cup organic basil
2 large cloves garlic (1 if you like it milder)
¼ cup rice parmesan or vegan parmesan*
¼ cup pine nuts (optional)
Salt to taste

Directions:
Put into a mixer and blend until smooth.

*Vegan parmesan contains soy, so I'm not a fan; but, it will work if you can't have rice or the tiny bit of dairy that is in the rice cheese.

NOTE: I love this recipe because I adore pesto, and in the summer it's great to use in a pasta salad! To make a quick **pasta salad**, do this:
Prepare rice pasta.
Sauté some yellow and green squash with red onion.
Add sautéed vegetables to rice pasta and toss with pesto sauce.
Place in refrigerator to cool.

Tomato Relish
Preheat oven to 250°.

Ingredients:
2 large ripe tomatoes, peeled, seeded, drained, and chopped
1 small white onion, chopped
3 tbsp fresh cilantro, minced
1 tbsp ground cumin
1 pinch cayenne pepper
salt to taste

Directions:
Peeling Tomatoes:
Cut out the stem.
Drop tomatoes into boiling water for about 1 minute.
Remove from water with a slotted spoon and immediately drop into a bowl of cold water and ice cubes (to stop cooking process).
Peel should practically slide off easily with the help of a paring knife.

Place cumin on a sheet of foil and place in oven to toast. About 3 minutes. WATCH carefully to make sure it doesn't blacken and burn.
Toss the tomatoes with the

onion, cilantro, cayenne, and toasted cumin.

Season with salt

SEASONINGS

The following examples of seasonings containing no fat, starch or sugar:

McCormick Montreal Chicken,
McCormick Garlic Pepper,
McCormick Italian Seasoning,
McCormick Steakhouse Seasoning Grinder,
McCormick Italian Herb Seasoning Grinder,
McCormick Broiled Steak Seasoning Salt,
McCormick Rotisserie Chicken Seasoning,
McCormick Herb Chicken Seasoning Spice ,
Tony Chachere's Original Creole Seasoning,
Classic Soul Food Seasoning Salt Spice,
Classic Steak Seasoning Salt Spice,
Classic Poultry Seasoning,
Weber Grill Creations N'Orleans Cajun Seasoning

CHICKEN

Cajun Chicken Breast

Ingredients:
4 ounces organic chicken breast
Weber Grill Creations N'Orleans Cajun Seasoning
lettuce
¼ medium lemon
salt and pepper to taste

Directions:
Marinade chicken breast in Cajun Seasoning in refrigerator for 30 or more minutes.
Place on grill (low to medium flame).
Place on bed of lettuce.
Sprinkle with salt, pepper, and lemon juice to taste.

Chicken Nuggets

Ingredients:
4 organic boneless chicken breasts
2 eggs
¾ cup of almond flour
¾ cup of brown rice flour

2 tablespoons crushed fresh garlic
sea salt
pepper
paprika
dried parsley

Directions:
Combine nut flour, crushed fresh garlic, sea salt, pepper, paprika, and dried parsley flakes.
Beat eggs.
Dip bite-sized pieces of chicken in the beaten egg, and then roll in the nut-flour mixture.
Fry in olive oil.
NOTE: Cook anything with almond flour a little more slowly than you would do with regular flour so it doesn't burn.

Chicken Veggie Packets

From: Edna Shaffer in Quick Cooking
Preheat oven to 375°
Makes 4 servings.

Ingredients:
4 boneless skinless chicken breast halves, about 1 pound
½ pound asparagus (cut into 1 inch pieces)
1½ cups yellow zucchini (cut into small cubes)
1 cup frozen pearl onions, thawed
½ cup julienned sweet red pepper
¼ teaspoon pepper
1 teaspoon dried thyme

Directions:
Flatten chicken breasts to 1/2 inch thickness.
Place each chicken breast on a piece of heavy-duty foil, about 12"x12".
Layer asparagus, zucchini, onions, and red pepper on top of each piece of chicken and sprinkle with thyme and pepper.
Fold foil around chicken and vegetables and seal tightly.
Place on a baking sheet.
Bake at 375 F for 20 minutes or until chicken juices run clear.

Chicken and No Tomato Pasta Sauce
Preheat oven to 400°F

Ingredients
4 boneless skinless chicken breast halves, about 1 pound
1 package of brown rice linguini
1 jar of roasted red peppers
½ jar pitted black olives
5 cloves of garlic
¼ cup extra virgin olive oil
½ teaspoon Chili powder
1 teaspoon garlic powder
½ teaspoon ground cumin

¼ teaspoon oregano
¼ teaspoon paprika
1 teaspoon apple cider vinegar
salt and pepper to taste

Directions:
Coat garlic cloves (skins on) with a small amount of oil and salt.
Wrap garlic cloves in and roast for about 15-20 min at 400F.
Cut chicken into bite-sized pieces and start cooking in a pan with a bit of oil and all spices listed above.
Start to cook your pasta.
Place roasted garlic cloves, roasted peppers, black olives, garlic powder, cumin, oregano, and apple cider vinegar into a food processor and begin to puree.
Slowly drizzle in the olive oil while blending.
Drain your pasta when done.
Mix together pasta, chicken, and sauce. Enjoy!

Chicken Parm Minus the Cheese

Preheat oven to 350^{OF}

Ingredients:
1 pound of chicken breast
2 large tomatoes
fresh basil leaves
2 teaspoons dried basil
½ cup of minced onions
¼ red pepper (minced)
6 cloves of minced fresh garlic (more or less to taste)
sea salt and pepper to taste
extra virgin oil

Directions:
Season the chicken breasts with salt and pepper and dry basil leaves.
Drizzle some extra virgin olive oil in pan and par cook the breasts a little on each side
Remove par cooked breasts from oil and place them on a baking sheet.
In a separate pan, drizzle in extra virgin olive oil and add diced tomatoes, minced peppers, garlic, onion, salt and pepper, and dried basil. Cook tomato mixture until its contents are tender and the mixture has a sauce-like consistency.
Cut the fresh basil leaves into ribbons and add to the sauce at the end. Mix well.
Pour the tomato sauce on top of the breasts.
Bake at 350 for about 10 minutes or until done.

Sicilian Hens

Ingredients:
2 Cornish hens, thawed, halved
¼ cup toasted sliced almonds
3 tablespoons drained capers
3 tablespoons chopped fresh parsley
1 garlic clove, chopped
½ tsp paprika
2 tsp olive oil
¼ tsp salt
⅛ tsp pepper
chopped ripe olives

Directions:
In food processor fitted with metal blade, combine almonds, capers, parsley, garlic, paprika, oil, and salt and pepper. Process until finely chopped but not pureed.

Pat mixture onto all sides of Cornish hens.
Place on a rack in slow cooker (crock pot).
If all hens do not fit on rack, place 2 halves on rack; lightly cover with heavy-duty foil.
Arrange remaining halves on top of foil.
Cover and cook on LOW 7-8 hours.
Sprinkle with chopped olives.

MEAT

Meatballs -By Lauren Insco
Optional: Preheat oven to 350^{oF}

Ingredients:
2 lbs. ground beef
1 medium onion, finely chopped
¾ tsp. Celtic sea salt
⅛ tsp. pepper
2 eggs
⅓ cup rice bran
2 to 3 cloves minced garlic

Directions:
Mix all ingredients together well.
Shape into meatballs, about 1¼".
Fry in pan (do not need oil or anything really unless your meat is particularly lean) or bake in the oven at 350 till done.
Use meatballs over spaghetti squash with a good Candida recipe for sauce or over brown rice pasta.

Peppercorn Steak

Ingredients:
four 8 oz. lean beef steak pieces
30 whole peppercorns, cracked
⅓ teaspoon salt
1 large or 2 medium sweet onions

Directions:
Crack pepper by placing in a towel and striking it with a wooden mallet or rolling pin.
Moisten steaks with filtered water and then pat steaks with cracked pepper and salt.
Heat water into a nonstick pan.
Place steaks and sliced onion into the pan and brown 15 minutes.

Sloppy Joes

Ingredients:
1 lb. grass fed ground beef
2 tbs. olive oil
1 medium onion, chopped
1 medium green pepper, chopped
2 cloves garlic, minced
2 cups of your favorite tomato sauce
1 tablespoon chili powder
½ teaspoon cumin powder

Directions:
Brown ground beef and crumble in pan.
Drain off fat.
Add olive oil, onions, peppers, and garlic to pan and sauté until tender.
Continue cooking and add in tomato sauce and chili and cumin powders.
Serve hot

SALADS

Blended Salad

This is about the quickest to prepare out of all the vegetable salad recipes. Blending all the raw ingredients into very small pieces makes it much easier to chew and digest. It's a great way to get the cleansing benefits of raw vegetables into your diet if you aren't used to eating a lot of raw foods. It reminds me of gazpacho soup!

There are endless variations. Here is the one I make often.

Ingredients:
½ large cucumber
½ red or yellow bell pepper
1 medium tomato
3 leaves of romaine or butter lettuce, roughly chopped
1 slice of mild onion (Vidalia or sweet red onion is nice)
½ tablespoon of dried dulse seaweed (about 1/2 tablespoon)
juice of ½ lemon
sea salt (added to the finished salad)

Directions:
Coarsely chop all the vegetables, place in a food processor fitted with a double blade, add lemon juice and pulse until everything is chopped very fine, it will look like salsa! Spoon into a serving bowl, and sprinkle with sea salt to taste. You may like a drizzle of extra virgin olive oil as well, or some sliced avocado. I like it topped with a few spoonsful of tuna salad or salmon salad. Makes 1 serving.

Broccoli Salad with Sun-dried Tomatoes, Red Onion and Mustard Vinaigrette

This vegetable salad recipe is an immune system boost on a plate! It goes nicely with sautéed chicken breasts, grilled steaks, or simply seasoned fish and seafood.

Ingredients:
1 bunch broccoli – stems peeled, sliced into thin rounds, then into matchsticks, tops cut into bite-sized florets
½ cup marinated sun-dried tomatoes drained, oil reserved separately – tomatoes sliced into thin strips
1 small red onion – sliced into very thin wedges – soaked in

cold water for 30 minutes to mellow the flavor if desired and drained well
1/3 cup oil (start with the reserved sun-dried tomato oil, add more
extra virgin olive oil as needed)
¼ cup raw apple cider vinegar
2 tablespoons homemade mustard
½ teaspoon dried oregano
1 clove garlic – crushed and minced
Grey sea salt and freshly ground pepper to taste

Directions:
Blanch the broccoli florets and stems for 10 seconds in boiling water, drain and spread on a large plate or baking sheet. Immediately place in the refrigerator for 10 minutes to chill. When the broccoli has chilled, spin it dry if necessary and place in a mixing bowl. Add drained onion slices and sun-dried tomatoes. In a small bowl whisk together the apple cider vinegar, mustard, oregano, garlic, salt and pepper. Add oil slowly and whisk to emulsify. Pour over vegetables and toss well to combine. Allow salad to marinate for one hour before serving, serve chilled or at room temperature. Serves 4 – 6

Cole Slaw

This is based on my dad's old recipe (made with good old mayo out of a jar). It's light, lemony and perfect with mild white fish, grilled chicken or hamburgers.

Ingredients:
5 cups shredded green cabbage
½ cup homemade mayonnaise (recipe below)
2 tablespoons fresh lemon juice
1 teaspoon celery seeds
good grey sea salt and plenty of fresh ground pepper to taste

Directions:
Place cabbage in a mixing bowl, add remaining ingredients and toss well to combine. Taste and adjust seasonings. Serves 3 - 4

Napa Cabbage, Sweet Onion and Tomato Salad with Zesty Garlic Vinaigrette

There is no oil in the dressing for this salad, so it's a great match for fatty meats like roast lamb, or chicken legs.

Ingredients:
8 large Napa cabbage leaves – sliced in half lengthwise, and then into very thin slices

3 slightly under-ripe tomatoes – sliced in half, and then into half-moon slices
1 vidalia or sweet Maui onion – sliced into thin half moons
2 large cloves garlic – crushed and minced
1 teaspoon dry mustard powder
3 tablespoons raw apple cider vinegar
Grey sea salt and freshly ground pepper to taste

Directions:
In a small bowl, combine the garlic, mustard powder, apple cider vinegar, salt and pepper. Set aside. Place the Napa cabbage, tomatoes and onion slices into a mixing bowl. Pour the vinegar mixture over and toss well to combine. Serves 3 – 4

Variation: Substitute a handful of fresh mint leaves for the Napa cabbage, and serve with lamb or grilled shrimp.

Paleo Tuna Salad
Ingredients:
1 medium onion
2 stalks celery
Nutmeg, salt and pepper
Olive oil
2 cans plain tuna
⅓ cup finely chopped walnuts
⅓ - ¾ cup paleo mayo (depending on how creamy you like it)

Directions:
Chop up the onion and celery, then pan fry it in the olive oil, with some nutmeg, salt, and pepper. Put it in the refrigerator to cool, if you prefer cold salad. Drain the tuna (giving the tuna water to the cats, of course!), and mix all of the ingredients together. Makes 2 large servings or 4 small servings. Its yummy stuff and makes for a great weekend lunch. From: Charlotte Williams on Paleo Food list

Summer Tomato and Basil Salad

This is one of those vegetable salad recipes that goes with just about anything!

Ingredients:

1 lb ripe tomatoes – a colorful assortment is great – sliced
2 cloves garlic – crushed and minced
4 tablespoons extra virgin olive oil
a large handful of fresh basil leaves, julienned
Grey sea salt and freshly ground pepper to taste

Instructions:

Arrange sliced tomatoes on a large serving platter. Sprinkle the chopped garlic over the slices, and then drizzle on the olive oil. Add salt and pepper, top with the basil leaves and serve at once.
Variations: Substitute cilantro, chives or other herbs in place of the basil. Serves 3 – 4

Thai Cucumber Salad

Here's a great version of the oil-free ariety of vegetable salad recipes. It goes well with fish, chicken or grilled meats.

Ingredients:

2 medium cucumbers – sliced in half lengthwise, seeds removed if they are very large, sliced diagonally
1 small red onion – sliced into thin wedges – soaked in cold water for 30 minutes to mellow the flavor if you like, and drained well
1 small red bell pepper – seeded, quartered, and sliced diagonally into strips
1 small yellow pepper – seeded, quartered, and sliced diagonally into strips
½ cup chopped fresh cilantro
juice from one or two limes
3 or 4 drops liquid stevia extract or a generous pinch of dry powdered stevia leaves (optional)
Fish sauce or grey sea salt to taste

Directions:

Place the cucumber, peppers, onions and cilantro into a mixing bowl. Mix together the lime juice, stevia and fish sauce or salt in a small bowl. Pour over the vegetables and mix well. Serve at once. Serves 3 – 4
Variations: Add fresh tomato wedges. Add hot fresh chiles. Add some freshly grated ginger

juice. Substitute fresh Thai basil for the cilantro.

Quinoa & Cilantro Salad with Lemon & Garlic

Ingredients:
1 cup of dry quinoa (used prepared brown rice)
½ tsp. of sea salt
½ bunch cilantro, chopped
½ cup corn (I used 1 orange bell pepper, chopped)
½ cup parsley, chopped

For Dressing:

2-3 cloves garlic, minced
¼ cup freshly squeezed lemon juice
2 tblsp. Extra-virgin olive oil
1 tsp. sea salt

Directions:

Rinse quinoa well with warm water & drain, to remove the bitter saponin. Place in bowl and let soak for 12-24 hours in water (or used brown rice and skip the soaking procedure) at room temperature. Drain water into 1 cup measuring cup. Add to make 1 cup, or discard if more than 1 cup remains. Add salt to water in a pot. Bring to a boil, add quinoa, reduce heat to low, cover, and let simmer 15-20 minutes, until all the water is absorbed. Fluff into large salad bowl and allow to cool.

Prepare vegetables and dressing. Combine garlic, lemon juice, oil, and salt, and pour over quinoa and toss well. Wash and spin dry cilantro leaves and chop into bite-size pieces. Add cilantro, corn (bell pepper) and parsley to quinoa. Toss gently. Serve at room temperature or chilled. Makes 4 to 6 servings.

SEAFOOD

Garlic Shrimp

Ingredients:

¾ lb shrimp (ecologically farmed and anti-biotic free)
1 tablespoon olive oil
1 tablespoon fresh parsley (I used 1 tsp dried)
1 tablespoon lemon juice
6 - 8 cloves garlic minced 1/2 teaspoon Celtic Sea Salt
1/8 teaspoon pepper

Directions:

Heat the olive oil over medium heat. Add the garlic and sauté for1 minute. Add the shrimp (which is peeled and deveined). Sautee for 3 minutes. Add the lemon juice, parsley, salt, pepper and cook for an additional minute. Serve over spaghetti squash, shredded zucchini or rice pasta.

Seafood Gumbo

Ingredients:

4 oz. seafood (shrimp, scallops, lobster or whitefish)
1 clove, chopped garlic
⅛ teaspoon garlic powder
2 large chopped Roma tomatoes
⅛ teaspoon celery salt
¼ teaspoon onion salt
⅛ teaspoon ground cayenne
¼ teaspoon Creole seasoning
2 packets stevia

Directions:

Sauté seafood with chopped garlic over high heat until lightly browned. Add remaining ingredients and simmer on low heat for 15minutes

Simply Broiled Scallops

Ingredients:

4 oz. scallops
Garlic salt
Fresh lemon juice

Instructions:

Rinse scallops and place in a shallow baking pan. Sprinkle with garlic salt and lemon juice. Broil on medium 6 to 8 minutes. Do not overcook.

SOUPS & STEWS

Chicken Egg Drop Soup

Ingredients:

4 cups chicken stock or broth
4 eggs, well beaten
Salt and freshly ground white pepper, to taste
¼ cup chopped scallions, for garnish
2 tablespoons chopped cilantro leaves, for garnish

Directions:

In a saucepan over high heat, bring the chicken stock or broth to a boil. Season with salt and pepper. With the soup boiling, pour in the beaten eggs in a thin, steady stream. Cook for about 2 minutes, until the egg is set. Ladle into 4 bowls and garnish with the scallions and cilantro.

Millet Stew

Ingredients:

1 cup millet
4 cups water
2 onions - cut in wedges
2 potatoes - cut in large chunks
2 carrots - cut in large slices
1 cup celery - cut in large slices
½ pound mushrooms - chopped
2 bay leaves
½ teaspoon basil
½ teaspoon thyme

Instructions:

Toast millet in dry skillet for about 5 minutes. Stir constantly to prevent burning. Add all ingredients to crock pot and cook 4 hours at high or 8 hours at low.

Chicken Escarole Soup

Ingredients:
2 cups chicken stock
2 cups water
1 Boneless skinless chicken breast (about ½ lb)
2 medium carrots; chopped
2 medium stalks celery; chopped
1 medium Onion; chopped
¼ cups minced parsley
⅛ teaspoon pepper
½ lb escarole, trimmed
1 small tomato; cored, seeded and chopped

Instructions:
In a large heavy saucepan over medium heat, bring the chicken stock and water to a simmer. Add the chicken, carrots, celery, onion, parsley and pepper. Cover and cook until the chicken is tender, about 20 minutes. Remove the chicken and set aside to cool. Stir in the escarole and tomato and simmer, uncovered, 5 -10 minutes until the escarole is tender. When the chicken is cool enough to handle, cut into ½ inch pieces, return to the saucepan and reheat, about 1 minute.

Chicken Poaching

Ingredients:
6 cups chicken stock
1 yellow onion finely chopped
2 carrots, peeled, halved lengthwise, and thinly sliced
2 celery stalks, thinly sliced
2 zucchini, thinly sliced
2 tablespoons finely chopped fresh parsley
2 oz of yeast, wheat and gluten free noodles
½ cup shredded or cubed, skinless cooked chicken meat
salt and freshly ground pepper

Instructions:
In a large saucepan over medium-low heat, bring the chicken stock to a simmer. Add the onion, carrots and celery and continue to simmer until the vegetables are slightly soft, about 10 minutes. Add the zucchini and 1 tablespoon of the parsley and cook until the zucchini is just tender, about 10 minutes longer. Add the noodles and simmer until they are just tender, 3-4 minutes, or according to the package directions. Three minutes before the noodles are done, add the chicken and heat through. Season to taste with salt and pepper. Ladle into warmed soup bowls and

sprinkle the tops with the remaining 1 tablespoon parsley. Serve immediately.

Curried Celery Soup – from Body Ecology Diet

Ingredients:

2 tablespoons Ghee
1 onion, chopped
1 leek, washed and sliced
1½ pounds celery, chopped
1 tablespoon medium or hot curry powder (or more to taste!)
3 large red-skinned potatoes
3¾ cups water or vegetable stock
1 bouquet garnir (Place a bay leaf, a sprig of thyme and a sprig of parsley on one piece of green leek. Cover with the remaining piece of green leek. Tie securely with fine string, leaving a length of string attached so that the bouquet garnie can be easily retrieved. Voila!)
2 tablespoons finely chopped mixed fresh herbs
Celtic Sea Salt and Herb-a-mare
Celery seed and celery leaves to garnish

Directions:

Heat the ghee in a large saucepan. Add the onion, leek and celery, cover and cook gently for about 10 minutes, stirring occasionally. Add the curry powder and cook for 2 minutes more, stirring occasionally. Add the potatoes, stock (or water) and bouquet garnircover and bring to a boil. Simmer for 20 minutes, until the vegetables are tender. Remove and discard the bouquet garnir and set the soup aside to cool slightly. Puree in a blender or food processor until smooth. We use a hand-held blender. Add the mixed herbs, season to taste and process VERY briefly. Return to the saucepan and reheat gently until piping hot. Ladle into soup bowls and garnish each
with a sprinkling of celery seeds and some celery leaves.

Roasted Red Pepper and Garlic Soup

Ingredients:

10 cloves garlic, minced
2 cans (16oz.each) red roasted peppers, diced
1 gallon chicken stock
½ cup butter
½ cup flour
2 teaspoons dried rosemary, crumbled

Salt and pepper, to taste

Directions:
In a large pot melt the butter and stir in the flour to make a roux. Cook the roux for about 7-10 minutes to get the flour taste out. Add the garlic. Pour in the chicken stock and bring to a boil; let thicken. Turn down the heat and add the diced red peppers and salt and pepper then add the crumbled rosemary.

SIDE DISHES

Black-Eyed Peas and Brown Rice

From
www.cleaneatingmag.com

Ingredients:
cups cooked, cold, long-grain brown rice
1 ¼ cups water
1 onion, chopped
2 celery stalks, chopped
2 garlic cloves, minced
¼ teaspoon freshly ground pepper
3 cups cooked black-eye peas
1 butternut squash, about 1 lb., peeled, seeded and cut into cubes
1 red bell pepper, stemmed, seeded and finely chopped
½ teaspoon red pepper flakes

Directions:
Put rice in a large bowl. Gently separate the grains and break apart any lumps. In a large frying pan, bring the water, onion, celery, garlic and pepper to a boil, stirring frequently. Add the black-eyed peas and squash and return to a boil, again stirring frequently. Reduce to low, cover and simmer, stirring occasionally, until the peas and squash are tender and most of the water has evaporated, about 20 minutes. Add the rice, bell pepper and hot pepper sauce. Simmer, stirring and tossing frequently until heated through, about 5 minutes. To serve, transfer to a bowl.

Homemade Applesauce

Ingredients:

apples (Granny Smith only)
1 teaspoon fresh lemon juice
½ cup water
1 packet stevia
½ teaspoon cinnamon

Instructions:

Peel, core and chop apples. Cook apples and water in a crock pot on low for 2 hours. When cooled, puree apples in blender while adding Stevia and cinnamon. Divide into 5 equal portions (usually about ½ cup per serving)

Desserts

Avocado Mousse

Ingredients:

2 avocados
½ cup organic strawberries
½ cup organic blueberries
2 tablespoons of nut butter
1 cup unsweetened almond milk

Directions:

Mix thoroughly in blender on high. Pour into bowl and place in refrigerator. Serve as mousse.

Apple Salad

Ingredients:

1 apple, cut into fine slices
1 teaspoon chopped fresh mint
1 tbsp. fresh lemon juice

Directions:

Mix together and serve.

Apple Berry Crumble

Preheat oven to 375°F

Ingredients:

5 organic Granny Smith apples, cored, peeled and sliced
1 cup organic blueberries
tablespoons coconut oil
3 cups ground almonds or almond meal
½ teaspoon cinnamon

Directions:

Sauté apples and blueberries in a pan with 2 tablespoons of coconut oil until fruit is softened. In separate bowl combine almonds meal, cinnamon and remainder of coconut oil to create the crumble. Pour the sautéed fruit into a pie tin and top with the crumble. Cook in preheated oven at 325 degrees for 30 minutes. Serve warm.

Candida Shortbread Cookies
By Lauren Insco
Preheat oven to 350°F

Ingredients:
1 cup brown rice flour
tablespoons virgin coconut oil, partially melted
¾ teaspoon stevia powder
½ teaspoon Celtic sea salt
1 egg
1 teaspoon vanilla flavoring (no alcohol)
2 tablespoon water
Directions:
Combine ingredients in mixing bowl; mix well. Drop by spoonsful onto greased baking pan. They will cook in the shape you put them in, so I flatten them slightly with a spoon. Bake for 10 – 14 minutes at 350. They will not brown because of the rice flour, so keep an eye on them. They are done if they bounce back when you touch one (use the tip of a utensil – not your finger!) Cool on rack. I always double this recipe, and freeze them in individual wrapped packets, so I can have a cookie whenever I'm in the mood for one. I am going to try modifying this recipe with some unsalted butter and see what that does, but the cookie does have a nice texture, like shortbread.
For a variation, I used these cookies to make peanut butter & jelly...I put a little almond butter in a bowl and mixed with a tiny bit of stevia. I spread it on a cookie and put some fresh raspberries on it....it was delicious! Tasted like peanut butter & jelly. It was so filling, I could only eat 1 cookie with 3 raspberries and about 1 or 2 tblsp. of almond butter, and I was done.

Carob Chip Cookies
Preheat oven to 375°F

Ingredients:
1 stick butter softened
¼ teaspoon stevia extract powder
1 egg
½ teaspoon vanilla
½ cup whole wheat flour
½ teaspoon salt
½ teaspoon baking soda 1 cup rolled oats
¼ cup chopped nuts
½ cup unsweetened carob chips

Directions:
Mix together the first four ingredients. Add the remaining ingredients in order with slight variations possible. Divide into

cookies and bake 10 min at 375 degrees F.

Carob Chip Oatmeal Cookies
(No white Flour)
Preheat oven to 350°F

Ingredients:
1 egg
½ teaspoon Stevia powder concentrate
2 packages of artificial sweetener (like Equal, Twin)
½ cup butter
½ teaspoon vanilla
1 cup oats
One third of a cup whole wheat flour
One third of a cup millet flour
½ teaspoon baking soda
Two thirds of a cup unsweetened carob chips

Directions:
Beat together first 5 ingredients. Add in flours, soda and oats. Mix well. Add in carob chips. Divide into cookies and bake 10-12 mins at 350 degrees F. Makes about 12-14 cookies. Optional: add cinnamon and/or nuts

Cashew Cake Batter
Ingredients:
1 cup cashews (soak first).
1¼ cup almond milk
a dash of sea salt
½ teaspoon alcohol-free vanilla extract
3 drops of Stevia
2 tablespoons coconut butter

Directions:
Blend, Refrigerate, sprinkle with cinnamon and enjoy!

Chewy Gluten Free/Low Sugar Cookie
Recipe courtesy Alton Brown, 2007
Preheat oven to 350°F

Ingredients:
Dry:
11 ounces brown rice flour, approximately 2 cups
½ ounce tapioca flour, approximately 2 tablespoons
1 teaspoon xanthan gum
1 teaspoon kosher salt
1 teaspoon baking soda

Wet:
8 ounces unsalted butter, room temperature
2 tablespoons of Coconut Oil (Melt with the butter)
1 cup Agave
1 cup light brown sugar
2 eggs
1 1/2 teaspoons vanilla extract
1 ½ cups semisweet chocolate chips, or less if you want to cut back on the sugar

Directions:

In a medium bowl, sift together dry ingredients the rice flour, cornstarch, tapioca flour, xantham gum, salt, and baking soda. Set aside. Melt the butter in microwave or in the bottom of small saucepan over low heat. Once melted, pour into the bowl of a stand mixer. Add both of the sugars to the bowl with the butter and using the paddle attachment, cream together on medium speed for 1 minute. Add the whole egg, egg yolk, milk and vanilla extract and mix until well combined. Slowly incorporate the flour mixture until thoroughly combined. Add the chocolate chips and stir to combine. Chill the dough in the refrigerator until firm, approximately 1 hour. Shape the dough into 2-ounce balls and place on parchment-lined baking sheets, 6 cookies per sheet. Bake for 9 to 10 minutes. Remove from the oven and cool the cookies on the pans for 2 minutes. Move the cookies to a wire rack and cool completely. Store cooked cookies in an airtight container.

Cinnamon Apple Zucchini Bread

Preheat oven to 325°F

Ingredients:

3 cups organic brown rice flour
1 teaspoon salt
1 teaspoon baking soda
1 teaspoon baking powder
3 teaspoon ground cinnamon
3 eggs
1 cup coconut oil
2 cups unsweetened applesauce
½ teaspoon stevia
3 teaspoon vanilla extract
2 cups grated zucchini
1 cup chopped walnuts (optional)

Directions:

Grease and flour two 8 x 4 inch pans w/ unsalted butter. Sift flour, salt, baking powder, baking soda, cinnamon, and stevia together in a bowl. Beat eggs, oil, and vanilla together in a large bowl. Beat in applesauce. Slowly add sifted ingredients and beat well. Stir in zucchini and nuts (if desired) until well combined. Pour batter into prepared pans and bake for 40 to 60* minutes, or until tester inserted in the center comes out clean. Do not over bake. Cool in pan on rack for 20 minutes. Remove bread from pan, and completely cool. *Note: I baked for 45 min. and it was perfect.

Coconut Cookies

Preheat oven to 350°F

Ingredients:

¼ cup coconut oil
1 teaspoon stevia
1 teaspoon organic vanilla extract
1 ¼ cups ground almonds or almond meal
½ cup desiccated coconut
¼ teaspoon salt
¼ teaspoon gluten free baking powder

Directions:

Blend stevia, coconut oil and vanilla extract in a bowl. In another bowl blend the almond meal, salt, baking powder, and desiccated coconut. Blend the contents of both the bowls together along with a bit of water to soften. Make one inch balls and put them on a lined baking tray. Flatten the balls to cookies. Cook at 350 degrees for 10 minutes.

Festive Carrot Cookies

Preheat oven to 350°F

Ingredients:

½ cup rice bran
½ cup almond meal
2 small zucchini, scrubbed, peeled, and finely chopped
1/4 cup Easy Clarified Butter, melted (melted butter with the white foamy stuff on top scooped off. The white stuff is the sugar part of butter)
2 tablespoons 100% Pure Vegetable Glycerin (usually found in the cosmetic section of health food stores doesn't affect blood sugar in ways that regular sugar does)
Stevia – (used 15 drops I it needs a little more)
1 large egg
½ cup chopped or ground fresh pecans (optional)
1 teaspoon vanilla (optional) (used the kind without alcohol)
¼ teaspoon sea salt (optional) (used almost a ½ tsp. Celtic sea salt)
2 teaspoon ground cinnamon

Directions:

Preheat oven to 350 degrees F. Place all ingredients in a large bowl; mix well. Place spoonfuls on a non-stick cookie sheet. Flatten with back of spoon. Bake 10-12 minutes. Approx 6 carbs each. (I cooked longer)

Hazelnut Blueberry Muffins
Preheat oven to 325°F

Ingredients:
1 egg
⅔ cup unsweetened applesauce
⅜ teaspoon stevia
¼ cup salted butter (softened)
two thirds cup soy milk
1½ cups brown rice flour
½ cup hazelnut flour/hazelnut meal
2½ tsp baking powder
1 teaspoon vanilla
1 cup blueberries
¼ cup chopped hazelnuts for topping (optional)

Directions:
In a medium bowl, sift flours, salt, baking powder and sugar until combined. In a separate large bowl beat butter, egg, milk, vanilla, and lemon zest. Gradually beat in flour mix. Mix until ingredients are just well-mixed. Fold in blueberries. Fill each greased or paper-lined muffin tin ¾ full will mixture. Sprinkle each muffin with chopped hazelnuts. Bake at 350 for 20-25 min.
Cool completely.

Hazelnut Cake
Preheat oven to 350°F

Ingredients:
2 cups ground hazelnuts
⅓ cup cocoa
1 teaspoon baking powder
¼ teaspoon salt
eggs
1 stick butter, melted
1 teaspoon vanilla
Artificial sweetener equivalent to 1 cup sugar
½ cup water

Directions:
Grease a 8 or 9" round pan or spring form pan or use cupcakes tins. Mix together the dry ingredients. Mix wet ingredients together add to dry. Pour and bake. The exact time will vary with the pan.

Oatmeal Cinnamon Carob Chip Cookies
Preheat oven to 325°F

Ingredients:
1 ½ cups brown rice flour
1 cup rolled oats
½ tsp stevia
½ cup butter (softened)
1 cup unsweetened apple sauce
1 egg
½ tsp baking powder
½ tsp baking soda
½ tsp vanilla extract
¼ tsp cinnamon
1 carob bar (broken into small chunks)
1 cup carob chips

Directions:
In a medium bowl, sift brown rice flour, cinnamon, and oats. In a separate large bowl, beat butter, unsweetened applesauce, and stevia until mixed well. Beat in egg, baking powder, baking soda, and vanilla. Gradually beat in sifted flour mix until mixed well. Stir in carob bar chunks and chips. Note: Batter will be slightly runny. Spoon onto parchment paper-lined cookie sheet and bake 10-14 minutes. Do not over bake. Cool completely on wire rack.

Olive Oil Almond Cake

Preheat oven to 350°F

Ingredients:
6 egg whites -
1 ¼ cups almond flour
¾ cup sweetener
1 teaspoon baking powder
2 teaspoon butter melted
teaspoons olive oil
½ teaspoon almond extract

Directions:
Mix egg whites till stiff and fluffy with 2 tsp. equivalent sugar substitute. Mix dry ingredients. Fold egg whites into dry ingredients. Melt butter. Add almond extract. Add to dry mix. Add oil. Makes 6-8 cupcakes or put into buttered cake pan (maybe with parchment paper). Bake at 350 till light brown on top and/or toothpick comes out dry.

Mum's Plain Pecan Apple Bread

Preheat oven to 355°F

Ingredients:
1 egg, beaten
2 cups almond flour
½ cup pecan flour
2 ripe apples, cooked and pureed
1 teaspoon baking soda
¼ teaspoon salt

Directions:
Beat all ingredients together. Pour into a long and narrow loaf tin, lined with paper and well-greased with butter or olive oil. Bake at 355 F for 15 minutes then at 320 degrees F for half an hour or until middle of loaf springs back when lightly pushed.

Pie Recipe

Preheat oven to 350°F

Low Carb Pie Crust Ingredients:

tablespoons of butter, melted
3 tablespoons of cream cheese, softened
¼ teaspoon salt
2 cups of almond flour
2 tablespoons of ground flax
1 egg yolk
¼ teaspoon vanilla or almond extract
⅛ teaspoon cinnamon
2 Splenda packets

Fruit Filling Ingredients:

pints berries
2 tablespoons ground Tapioca (you can use instant tapioca)
packets of Splenda
2 tablespoons butter
one eighth teaspoon nutmeg
Juice of a half a lemon
Grated rind of a half a lemon

Directions:

Mix pie crust ingredients. Press into pan. Bake at 350 till slightly brown. Pour fruit filling into crust and bake 350 for approx 45min to 1 hour.

Pumpkin Poundcake

Preheat oven to 300°F

Ingredients:

3 cups almond flour
1 teaspoon stevia. Use depending on desired sweetness.
1½ teaspoon baking powder (aluminum free
3 teaspoons pumpkin pie spice
½ teaspoon nutmeg
¼ teaspoon ground cloves
½ teaspoon sea salt
7 Eggs
1½ cups canned pure organic pumpkin
1½ teaspoon vanilla (no alcohol)

Directions:

Spray loaf pan (9x5) with spray or wipe down with coconut oil. In a bowl, whisk together the almond flour, Stevia, baking powder, pie spice, and salt. In another bowl, beat the eggs and the whisk in the pumpkin and vanilla. Combine the dry and wet ingredients and stir until combined. Pour the batter into the prepared pan. Bake until golden brown in color and a toothpick comes out clean when stuck in the middle. This takes about 1½ hours. Cool completely before removing from the pan. Slice into 12 slices.

Strawberries and Crème

Ingredients:
Hand full of small-medium strawberries
1 T. milk
1 drop Vanilla Crème Stevia
1 packet stevia

Directions:
Slice strawberries and toss with packet of stevia to taste. Measure milk into separate bowl and stir in liquid stevia. Pour over strawberries.

Vanilla Almond Coconut Sugar Cookies
Preheat oven to 350°F

Ingredients:
¾ cup unsweetened applesauce
½ teaspoon stevia
½ cup butter (softened)
one third cup soymilk (could substitute hemp milk or almond milk)
2 teaspoons vanilla
¾ cup brown rice flour
one third cup coconut flour
2 teaspoons potato starch
½ teaspoon baking powder
½ teaspoon baking soda
½ cup sliced almonds

Directions:
In a large bowl, beat unsweetened applesauce, butter, and Stevia for 2 minutes until well-creamed. Add vanilla and soymilk and beat for an additional minute. In a separate bowl, mix together dry ingredients except almonds. Add dry mix to wet mix and briefly mix, then add almonds. Continue mixing until just blended. The batter should have a moist and fluffy consistency.
Spoon onto parchment paper-lined cookie sheet and bake 10-14 min. Do not over bake. Cool completely on wire rack.

Vanilla Custard
Preheat oven to 325°F

Ingredients:
2 cups Vanilla Rice Dream or milk
3 eggs
12 drops Stevia extract

Directions:
Heat milk and Stevia (just to boiling in medium saucepan). Let cool 5 or so minutes (you don't want the milk too hot or it will cook the eggs!). Beat eggs, vanilla and salt in large

bowl until smooth. Gradually beat in hot milk. Pour mixture into 5 custard cups or 1 quart glass casserole; sprinkle generously with nutmeg (optional). Place custard cups or casserole in roasting pan; add 1-inch hot water to roasting pan. Bake, uncovered,
1 teaspoon vanilla extract
one eighth teaspoon salt
Ground nutmeg (optional)

in preheated 325*F (160*C) oven until sharp knife inserted halfway between center and edge of custard comes out clean, 45 to 60 minutes. Remove custard dishes from roasting pan; cool on wire rack. Refrigerate until chilled. Makes 5 servings.

Drinks

Almond Milk

Ingredients:
1 cup raw almonds (or blanched, if available)
cups warm water
¼ teaspoon steviaPlus
1 teaspoon vanilla
½ teaspoon almond extract (optional)

Directions

To blanch almonds:
Place the almonds into a microwave-safe bowl and pour in enough water to cover them. (This is additional water, NOT the 4 cups referenced above.) Microwave on high power for 2 to 3 minutes. The skins on the almonds should become loose and peel easily. Remove and discard the skins.

To make milk:
Place blanched almonds in a blender container and discard the blanching water.
Pour the 4 cups warm water into blender container and begin to process water and almonds on low speed, gradually turning the speed up to high.
Blend the almonds and water on high speed until completely smooth, about 3 to 4 minutes.
Turn the blender off. Add the remaining ingredients and blend again until combined.

Place a clean towel, cheese cloth, or paper towel into a strainer placed over a large bowl.
Pour the almond milk into the cloth-lined strainer.
Allow the mile drain completely and press out as much excess liquid as possible.
Pour the milk into a pitcher and store it in the refrigerator for up to two weeks.
You may want to stir it every day to keep the oils from separating.

Frozen Cappuccino

Ingredients:
1 cup crushed ice
drops English Toffee stevia
1 tablespoon milk
drops clear stevia
5 drops Vanilla Crème stevia

Directions:
Mix in blender until smooth.
Pour into glass and serve.

Hot Chocolate

Ingredients:
8 oz hot water
5 drops Chocolate stevia
2 drops Vanilla Crème stevia

Directions:
Mix and serve

Hot Raspberry Chocolate

Ingredients:
8 oz. hot water
drops Chocolate Raspberry stevia
3 drops Vanilla Crème stevia

Directions:
Mix and serve

Strawberry Lemonade

Ingredients:
½ cup crushed ice
1 cup water
1 tablespoon fresh lemon juice
3 oz. fresh or partially defrosted strawberries
25 drops lemon flavored stevia
10 drops clear stevia

Directions:
Mix in blender until smooth.
Pour into glass and serve or freeze to make shaved ice.

Additional Recipes

Quinoa

I've only recently discovered Quinoa, and I think I'm going to be hooked on it! It's very easy to prepare and has a lot of protein and calcium which we all need.

Ingredients:
¼ cup quinoa
½ cup of water
½ green apple

Directions:
Rinse quinoa (as you would rice)
Place in rice cooker with 1.5 times the amount of water.
Cook approximately 20 minutes or until the quinoa has the consistency of a firm cooked rice.
Add slices of green apple to cooked quinoa.
Drizzle with honey if you like._It should be ready within 20 mins! Yum!

Fried Rice

Ingredients:
1 cup brown rice, already cooked
2 eggs
½ cup of peas and corn
1 medium carrot, chopped
1 small cucumber, chopped
salt & pepper to taste

Directions:
Warm a skillet.
Add already-cooked rice and stir until any clumps are removed.
Push rice to edges of skillet to form a clear space in the middle.

Break the eggs into the middle of the rice.
Allow eggs to heat for 10-15 seconds before starting to stir.

You want the eggs scrambled, but not mixed in with the rice.
Add a little bit of salt and pepper.
Add peas and corn and carrot.
Keep stirring the mixture until the eggs are cooked and the rice is warmed up.
Turn off skillet just as egg is cooked. Serve!

Veggie Egg Scramble

Ingredients:
3 eggs
¼ of a tomato, chopped
3 small mushrooms, chopped
1 avocado, sliced
¼ cup chopped cucumber
¼ cup chopped carrot
tomato sauce (optional)

Directions:
Break eggs into a heated skillet.
Wait 10-15 seconds or until eggs start to cook to start stirring.
Keep stirring the eggs to scramble them.
Take eggs out of the skillet just before they are completely cooked (eggs should be a bit fluffy and soft still).
Place eggs onto a plate and top with raw chopped tomato, mushrooms, cucumber, and carrot.
Add slices of avocado to taste.
Pour tomato sauce over all as desired.

Herb Pork Chops

Ingredients:
boneless pork loin chops, cut 3/4 inch thick
4 teaspoons lemon juice
½ teaspoon dried thyme or savory, crushed
½ teaspoon dried marjoram or basil, crushed
¼ teaspoon ground ginger

Directions:
Trim fat from chops.
Brush both sides of chops with lemon juice.
Stir together thyme, marjoram, and ginger.
Rub herb mixture onto both sides of chops.
Place chops on the unheated rack of a broiler pan.
Broil 3-4 inches from the heat for 4 – 5 *min per-side* or until no pink remains and juices run clear. Turn once.

Pork Chop & Vegetable Skillet

Ingredients:
1 deboned, thick pork chop
¼ cup beef bouillon
1 medium potato, halved lengthwise
2 medium carrot
½ green bell pepper, cut in chunks
salt and pepper

Directions:
Brown the pork chop in small amount of oil over medium heat.

Push chop to the side of the skillet and add the bouillon, potato, and carrot.
Place green pepper chunks on the pork chop.
Season everything with salt and freshly ground pepper.
Cover and simmer for about 45 minutes until the vegetables and chop are tender.
Add more bouillon if necessary.

Meat Marinade

Ingredients:
1 large clove garlic
2 tablespoons lemon juice
1 tablespoon raw unpasteurized apple cider vinegar*
1½ teaspoon steak spice
½ teaspoon celery salt
2 tablespoons oil
½ teaspoon salt

*Vinegar-containing foods are allowed on the Candida diet when well heated and eaten hot.

Directions:
Mix all ingredients together being sure the meat is well coated. I have used this to marinade chicken breasts and on pork ribs in the crock pot.

Chicken Stock

Ingredients:
2½ quart water
1 pound chicken bones or carcass of roasted
3½lb chicken
1 yellow onion, cut up
1 celery stalk, cut up
1 carrot, peeled and cut up
2 fresh flat-leaf (Italian) parsley sprigs
½ teaspoon salt
½ teaspoon dried thyme
¼ teaspoon peppercorns
1 bay leaf

Directions:
In a stock pot over medium-high heat, combine the water and chicken and bring slowly to a boil.
Skim off any fat and detritus that rises to the surface.
Add onion, celery, carrot, parsley, salt, thyme, peppercorns, and bay leaf.
Reduce the heat to medium and simmer uncovered for 2 hours.
Check from time-to-time, and skim off fat and detritus that appears on the surface.
Remove from the heat and let cool for 15 minutes.
Strain through a fine-mesh sieve into a large bowl and use

immediately or let cool, cover, and refrigerate for up to 5 days or freeze for up to 1 month Before using, remove and discard any fat congealed on top.

Rice Milk (requires a blender)

Ingredients:
1 cup dry brown rice
cups water
1 ¼ cup of almonds
1 teaspoon vanilla extract (optional)

Directions:
Mix rice, almonds, and water and let soak at room temperature for at least 4 hours or in the refrigerator overnight. (I put rice, almonds, and water right into the blender container and place that in the refrigerator.)
Blend rice and water in blender on high for about 1 minute.
Strain out rice from water (save water solution).
Add vanilla, blend again.
Refrigerate.
Because you do not strain it there will be some fiber, but they will soon sink to the bottom and you simply drink the top.

Some days, when you're over with Candida you might want to add frozen fruit and stevia or Splenda™ to obtain a nice milk shake.

Pumpkin Cookies
Preheat oven to 350°F

Ingredients:
1½ cups Quinoa Flour
½ teaspoon salt
1 teaspoon baking soda
3 tablespoons plus one teaspoon Truvia™ (stevia)
1 tablespoon Cinnamon (or more)
dash of ground clove
nutmeg (if desired)
½ cup unsalted butter
2 eggs
1 cup pumpkin
Pecans to taste

Directions:
Combine dry ingredients.
Combine butter and eggs and pumpkin in large bowl.
Add dry ingredients to the wet ingredients. Incorporate nuts.
Place tablespoon size drops on cookie sheet.
Bake 350 for 10-12 minutes.

Pumpkin Pie Pudding

Ingredients:
60 ounces of canned pumpkin
(plain pumpkin, not pie mix)
¾ cups quinoa flour
3 eggs
1½ cup almond or coconut milk
2 rounded tablespoons of
Truvia™
1 teaspoon vanilla
cinnamon to taste
ground clove to taste
Salt to taste
nutmeg to taste

Directions:
Place all ingredients in a large slow cooker.
Cook about 7 hours on low.
Let cool before placing in refrigerator.
Top with whipped cream that is sweetened with Truvia™ (stevia). This lasts in the refrigerator for at least a week. It makes a huge batch, but you can cut the recipe in half.

Veggie Chili (but adding cooked beef to it is yummy, too!) (Adapted from Taste of Home Magazine)

Ingredients:
medium zucchini, chopped
2 medium onions, chopped
1 large green pepper, chopped
1 large red pepper, chopped
cloves of chopped fresh garlic
¼ cup olive oil or grapeseed oil
56 ounces Italian stewed tomatoes, chopped. Save the juice
15 ounces canned tomato sauce
15 ounces canned pinto beans
15 ounces canned black beans
15 ounces canned kidney beans
2 chopped jalapeno peppers
½ cup chopped cilantro
¼ cup chopped parsley
2 tablespoons chili powder
2 teaspoons stevia
1 teaspoon kosher salt
3 teaspoons ground cumin
A dash of cinnamon if desired

Directions:
Sauté zucchini, onions, green and red peppers and garlic in oil until tender. Stir in the tomatoes with the reserved juice. Add tomato sauce, beans, jalapenos, and seasonings.
Bring to a boil over medium heat.
Reduce heat. Cover and simmer for at least 30 minutes stirring occasionally. This tastes better after it sits in the refrigerator for a day or so.

Butternut Squash and Chiles

Ingredients:
2 tablespoons grapeseed oil
1 ½ cup chopped onion
1 ½ to 2 pounds butternut squash, peeled, seeded and chopped into bite-sized pieces.
4-5 Poblano chilies peeled, charred over a flame or in broiler, placed in glass bowl, covered
salt to taste (1 tsp or so

Directions:
Heat oil in large sauté pan on med-high.
Add onions and cook about 3-4 minutes.
Add squash, salt, and chili powder. Stir.
Cover and cook until the squash is almost tender: about 10-12 minutes.
Stir in chilies and cook uncovered for 3 or so minutes.
Serve hot.

Posted by Tracey

Made in United States
North Haven, CT
10 July 2024

54629109R00143